COSMETIC SU...
AND BEAU...

The Cosmetic Surgery and Beauty Guide
Copyright © 1993
Edited by Trevor Lansdown
Published by Prowse & Saunders Ltd
The Studio Centre, Wiston Road,
Nayland, Colchester, Essex CO6 4LT
Telephone: 0206 262262
Origination: Anglia Photoset Ltd, Colchester.

All rights reserved. No part of this book may be reproduced, stored in a retrieval system or transmitted in any form or by any means, electronic, electrical, chemical, mechanical, optical, photocopying, recording or otherwise without prior written permission from the publishers.

Any opinions stated within the text of The Cosmetic Surgery and Beauty Guide 1993 are not necessarily those of the publishers. Any prices quoted may be subject to change without notice.

Acknowledgements
The publishers would like to thank the following for their advice and assistance during the preparation of this book:

The authors of Cosmetic Surgery – Andrew Skanderowicz FRCS and Edward Latimer-Sayer FRCS
Chrissie Painell – The Beauty Guide
Cosmetic Dentistry
The British Dental Health Foundation
Pamela Prowse – for being the best Mum

Picture sources:

Colchester Clinic of Cosmetic Surgery

B.A.C.S.

Beauty pictures. Léa 0836 549027

Front cover – Russell Walker

An Introduction to Cosmetic Surgery Techniques

Leading surgeons Edward Latimer-Sayer FRCS and Andrew Skanderowicz FRCS, from London's Highgate Private Hospital (View Road, London N6 4DJ) have compiled and written the following 'warts and all' operation descriptions. They have produced facts – not glamour about the cosmetic surgery business. And they speak plainly about pitfalls and risks. Operative techniques and general patient response are described in everyday language. Don't ask for Michelle Pfieffer's nose . . . it's already spoken for!

CONTENTS

Introduction	4
Foreword by Dr Hilary Jones	6
Factors Common to All Surgical Procedures	10
Pre-operative Considerations	11
Seeking Advice – Finding a Surgeon	12
Pre-operative Consultation & Counselling	14
The Routine Admission to a Clinic	15
The Causes of Disappointment	17
Anaesthesia	20
Facelift	23
The Lips	26
Eyelid Surgery	27
Treatment of Facial Lines and Wrinkles	28
Correction of Protruding Ears	32
Reshaping the Nose – Rhinoplasty	33
Chin Augmentation – Mentoplasty	34
Breast Augmentation (Enlargement)	38
Breast Uplift – Mastopexy	42
Breast Reduction	46
Gynaecomastia	48
Correction of Inverted Nipples	50
Body Contour Surgery – Liposuction	52
Abdominal Lipectomy – Tummy Tuck	54
Varicose Veins	56
Spider or Thread Veins	58
Removal of Tattoos	60
Scar Revision	62
The Treatment of Baldness	63
Correction of Muscle & Bony Defects	64
Skin Lumps & Bumps	65
A Profile on Cindy Jackson after 12 Operations	66
Cosmetic Dentistry	69
Health & Beauty with Chrissie Painell	74

COSMETIC SURGERY:

'This is the book for you', says Dr Hilary Jones

Cosmetic surgery is here to stay. The practice is enjoying rapid growth through popular demand and is now well and truly on the medical map. The British public has accepted it and long gone are the days when sceptics scoffed at the very idea – accusing people of being unduly vain, foolish, or both.

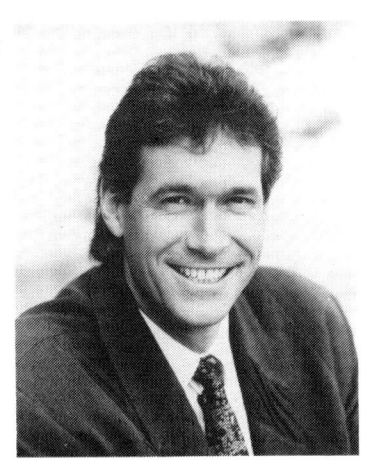

People have been attracted by the appeal of effective, safe and successful cosmetic surgery – and now they want to take advantage of it. Fortunes are spent on clothes and cosmetics – there's nothing new in the desire to look good and feel good – by whatever means.

Body contours can be altered, to some extent, by working out in the gym. And thanks to make-up, blemishes and wrinkles can be temporarily hidden or disguised – but success in these areas is limited.

Cosmetic surgery however, has the potential to 'make dreams come true' – to make someone truly happy with his or her appearance, possibly for the first time ever, and by giving the patient confidence and self-esteem that may have been lacking.

Changing the shape of a nose, the size of a breast, the reduction of facial lines, all come under the surgeon's remit.

Over the years in general practice I have seen at first hand how important inner well-being and psychological confidence really are.

Lack of esteem is typical in cases of depression. Poor confidence and the absence of ambition stem from anxiety and the negative feelings that come with self-doubt.

But if the feeling of self-worth can be boosted, often all those negative factors holding a person back can melt away.

As with medical advances, beauty treatments change all the time. They are frequently improved and updated. This guide offers the very latest information on how to tone up and look good, covering everything from brown lines to flaky fingernails; exfoliative massages to fruit facials. Pioneering developments in dentistry, like bleaching, procelain inserts and veneers, are all addressed on the following pages.

Modern techniques linked to superior surgical skills and sophisticated equipment can achieve more than ever before but cosmetic surgery, is not suitable for everyone. Prospective patients should remember that results with a scalpel can never by 100% guaranteed. Counselling and discussion prior to surgery are vital – as is selecting the most suitable surgeon for the job!

The Cosmetic Surgery and Beauty Guide 1993 plays its part in allaying the confusion that is still widespread through the media about the value and risks associated with cosmetic surgery.

It gives a sound, impartial and realistic overview of the subject and runs through every cosmetic operation currently routinely performed, including liposuction and face-lifts.

So if you're curious about the feasibility of 'finally going for the nose job' this is the book for you.

I highly recommend it and hope that anyone ever contemplating cosmetic surgery will read it – and that includes my patients!

On Face Value . . .

The number of people having cosmetic surgery has been steadily increasing over the past few years. They come from all walks of life and are of all ages. This increase is due to the public awareness of the benefits and the fact that such surgery is now socially acceptable. Furthermore, recent advances in the design of implants and surgical and anaesthetic techniques have greatly improved the results and shortened the time needed for recovery. Another reason for the rise in popularity of cosmetic surgery has been the increase in media coverage and publicity.

The aim of cosmetic surgery is to improve the appearance. It is important to stress that surgery is not an exact science and that the surgeon cannot always precisely match what a patient has in mind. Results are not guaranteed!

Most patients do not need cosmetic surgery in the medical sense, such as in the way that they might need to have their appendix removed. Cosmetic surgery is performed to please the patient. The test of success is not whether the patient lives or is relieved of symptoms, but whether he or she is pleased with the result. A good candidate for cosmetic surgery is, by definition therefore, a patient who is likely to be pleased. Nearly all patients who are good candidates are absolutely delighted!

The most common reason why people consider having cosmetic surgery is to look normal. They may feel that some part is too large or too small or does not fit in with the rest of themselves. They might also compare themselves to 'images of perfection' as portrayed in the media and sometimes they get teased or subjected to ridicule.

This desire to look 'normal' and to be accepted is extremely strong. In primitive societies, there are sometimes barbaric rituals that young people have to endure in order for them to become a full member of the tribe. In spite of this, they complete their ordeal with a sense of pride. Funnily enough, these often involve "cosmetic" surgery like body perforation using bones and bamboo. The result is that the initiate becomes recognizably part of the community. We don't go in for barbaric rituals in the Western world in the main. Nevertheless if someone looks very different from other members of a community they will find it much harder to fit in. To become an outcast from a community is one of the worst things that can happen to an individual. It has been for a long time a punishment for serious crimes.

This pressure to belong, and to look like everyone else, comes as much from within the person as it does from the community itself. A person who feels he looks different, but is confident enough to cope with it and put it the back of his mind does not have a problem. Many people have their confidence ruined by being self conscious of what they consider to be a blemish. Curiously, this is often only in the eye of the beholder. Other people may not even notice the blemish or might readily accept it.

THE CONFIDENCE FACTOR

A feeling of lack of confidence, and the hope that cosmetic surgery will provide that confidence, is the main reason, certainly for young people, to think about having something done. Nearly always, in response to the question "What are you hoping to get out of the operation" people will say that they want to feel more confident.

It is not just a psychological problem to be different. It's also difficult to get clothes that fit properly if you are very different from the usual shape and size. Manufacturers tend to cater best for the common sizes of clothes and shoes and this only adds to the sense of being unusual and isolated.

Sometimes people avoid particular activities because they draw attention to a feature that they normally hide easily. Many patients who hate their ears because they stick out don't like swimming. This is because wet hair exaggerates the problem. Some people don't like going on holiday because revealing clothes expose parts of themselves that they don't like!

The operations briefly described in this book have been performed successfully thousands of times throughout the world and most patients are very happy with the results of their surgery.

Occasionally reasons for having surgery bear little relationship to any physical problem, such as a wife trying to win back an errant spouse who has run off with a blonde. Cosmetic surgery is not the answer . . .

Factors Common to All Surgical Procedures

Every surgical procedure carries a small risk. This section deals with post operative events which can occur after any surgical operation.

PAIN AND DISCOMFORT: Surgical procedures result in discomfort for the patient. The degree and duration of this will depend on the nature of the operation and the patient's pain threshold. Tablets or injections are usually given in the immediate post operative period. Patients are discharged when they are comfortable.

SCARS: All surgical incisions heal with a scar. The surgeon tries to place incisions where they are not easily seen, such as in natural skin folds or behind the hairline. It is wrong to think that scars will be invisible or that they will fade to nothing in time. Wound healing is a complex process and scarring can be very variable. Most scars will look worse (red and raised) for some time after the operation before they mature and become pale. In general scars take 6–18 months to mature and there will always be a permanent mark, no matter how inconspicuous, where an incision has been made. Scars can occasionally be bad for no apparent reason and may require further treatment at a later stage. Complications such as infection or stretching of the wound can lead to bad scars. Some areas of the body and some skin types are notorious for producing worse scars than others.

BRUISING AND SWELLING: This is the body's natural response to injury. Every surgical procedure is followed by a period of bruising and swelling, depending on the nature and extent of the surgery.

BLEEDING AND HAEMATOMA: Sometimes bleeding can continue after the end of the operation or restart after an interval. It can either track to the surface, or more commonly, collect beneath the skin. Such a collection of blood is called a haematoma and if it becomes large enough it may require treatment.

INFECTION: A wound can become infected for a variety of reasons. Prompt and effective treatment is necessary to prevent further complications. Infections can also occur as a result of surgery in areas quite distant from the operation such as in the chest or urinary system.

DEEP VEIN THROMBOSIS: This is the situation in which blood has clotted in the deep veins of the calf. It is rare in patients undergoing elective cosmetic surgery. If the clot becomes dislodged and travels to the lungs it can have very serious consequences. Patients with a previous history of post operative deep vein thrombosis should warn the surgeon and the anaesthetist before the operation. Oral contraceptives increase the risk of deep vein thrombosis and there is some controversy about the benefit of stopping such treatment before surgery. It is thought wise to stop oral contraceptives prior to certain operations.

ALLERGIC REACTIONS TO DRUGS AND DRESSINGS: Various drugs are administered during the course of an operation particularly if there is a general anaesthetic. It is important to avoid giving any drug to a patient who might be allergic to it. Any known allergy must be reported to the surgeon and the anaesthetist before the operation. Severe allergic responses have to be dealt with promptly and effectively to avoid serious consequences.

BLOOD TRANSFUSION: This is seldom required in cosmetic surgery. All blood is carefully screened by the blood transfusion service for any infectious agent before it is released for use. It is quite common for patients to be given some fluid with a drip during and after operations.

DRAINS: Sometimes small flexible tubes are used to let out collections of blood or other fluids from a wound. They are removed a day or two after the operation.

Pre-operative Considerations

1. All patients are strongly encouraged to stop **smoking**. Smoking is not only a recognised health hazard in its own right but is responsible for a number of post operative problems and complications in patients who have a general anaesthetic.

a. Chest: Heavy smokers are more likely to develop a chest infection post operatively, particularly after major procedures.

b. Circulation: Heavy smokers are more liable to suffer the consequences of impaired circulation. This can lead to flap necrosis (loss of the skin resulting in bad scars) following a facelift or abdominoplasty.

2. **Alcohol an aspirin** should be avoided for two weeks before and after any significant operation. Both impair clotting and hence the patient is more likely to bleed during and after the operation.

3. **Abstinence from food and drink** from early morning or the previous midnight is essential depending on the time of the operation and the orders of the anaesthetist.

Seeking Advice – Finding a Surgeon

In Britain, specialist medical practitioners are forbidden to advertise their services to the public. This means that the average patient seeking cosmetic surgery will experience difficulty in finding the right surgeon to perform their operation unless he or she already knows of a surgeon who can help. Under the present system a patient can find a surgeon by one of three channels.

1. Be seeking a referral from their GP.
2. By recommendation from another patient.
3. By approaching one of the many clinics, agencies or advisory centres which advertise freely to the public.

THE GENERAL PRACTITIONER

This is the system of referral advocated by the General Medical Council. However many patients contemplating cosmetic surgery do not want to involve their GP. There are many reasons for this. Some do not wish to burden their overworked doctor with a problem involving vanity when he is already far too busy with genuine medical problems. Many fear that the GP's staff would not keep it a secret. Others are not registered with a GP. Some admit that they have little trust or faith in their GP and are too shy and embarrassed to approach him with such a delicate, personal and private problem. There are still a number of GPs who are less than enthusiastic about cosmetic surgery.

RECOMMENDATION FROM ANOTHER PATIENT

This is arguably the best way of being referred to a surgeon who has at least proved that he is competent at performing the procedure. Unfortunately not all patients will admit to their friends that they have had cosmetic surgery.

CLINICS WHICH ADVERTISE TO THE PUBLIC

In general terms, those which have been in existence for a number of years have stood the test of time. The reputation of a clinic depends largely on the reputation of the surgeon(s) employed. Unfortunately clinics may not divulge the name of the surgeon in advance of the consultation, but the prospective patient should determine that he is a Fellow of the Royal College of Surgeons (FRCS) and a member of a professional organisation, either The British Association of Cosmetic Surgeons or the British Association of Aesthetic Plastic Surgeons.

COSMETIC SURGERY AND THE NHS

The NHS does not readily cater for cosmetic surgery, priority being given to those patients with serious or life-threatening conditions. Most patients who have cosmetic surgery under the NHS have to wait a long time for treatment.

For additional information on the above named associations you can contact them by writing enclosing SAE specifying your requirements:

B.A.C.S., 17 Harley Street, London W1N 1DA.

B.A.A.P.S., Royal College of Surgeons, 35–43 Lincoln Inn Fields, London WC2A 3PN.

PRE-OPERATIVE CONSULTATION AND COUNSELLING

The results of cosmetic surgery can be very gratifying to both the patient and the surgeon. Before the patient has any treatment a consultation with the surgeon should take place and there should be a full discussion without any obligation. The importance of this consultation cannot be over-emphasized. All the patient's questions should be answered and the patient should be given time to think over what has been said and what has been proposed. A consultation is also essential because the surgeon has to ask the patient about their past medical history and health to find out if there are any details which might influence an operation. When the surgeon knows more about the patient he is in a better position to operate effectively and safely. The surgeon will normally communicate with the patient's GP after the consultation, as long as the patient allows him to.

At the initial consultation the surgeon has a duty to decide if the patient has a problem which can be improved by an operation. Sometimes a patient's feelings about what he or she looks like are very different from what other people can see. The best results in cosmetic surgery are obtained when the surgeon and the patient agree about the problem in the first instance. Then the surgeon has to ask himself whether there is an appropriate treatment which will improve it. It is obviously pointless to undertake a treatment which might not work or might even make things worse.

Once the surgeon has decided that there is a treatment which will work, he should fully inform the patient about the operation and the post operative course of events; when stitches are removed and when the patient can be seen in public again after the operation. Cosmetic surgery is not invisible mending, but by careful operative technique and the accurate positioning of incisions the scars can be almost invisible and only show on the closest examination. Patients should realise that some skin heals better than others and this of course should emerge in the initial consultation and be fully discussed. All likely complications should be discussed fully.

A patient who knows more above the operation because everything has been explained to them is more likely to be pleased with the result.

The surgeon himself should carry out the initial consultation, the surgery and all the post operative care and should be available to the patient at all times during the treatment process.

THE ROUTINE ADMISSION TO A CLINIC

Most patients are asked to attend the clinic quite early on the day of the operation or sometimes the night before in order that blood tests can be carried out. It is also to give the surgeon and anaesthetist a chance to see the patient and answer any last minute questions. A good margin of safety in the timing of the journey by public transport is essential to allow the patient to arrive at the clinic in good time without being stressed and hurried. After an operation it is a good idea if someone else takes the stress of driving.

Once at the clinic, most patients will undergo the admission procedure. Nurses will carefully fill out forms and will attach an identity bracelet to the patient. Blood and urine may be taken for routine tests. The nurses and the anaesthetist will make sure that the patient has not had anything to eat or drink for some hours before the operation if a general anaesthetic is to be given.

The patient will be asked to change out of their ordinary clothes and put on an operation gown. It is never a good idea to bring valuables to a clinic but rings, watches etc which will have to be removed before the operation should be entrusted to the nurses and put in a safe place. Patients should bring to the clinic toiletries enough to last them for the expected stay.

The anaesthetist will ask a series of questions concentrating on previous anaesthetics and illnesses relevant to the anaesthetic. Further medical tests may be arranged. If necessary the anaesthetist will order a sedative drug to be given an hour or so before the start of the operation.

Shortly before the operation, porters or nurses will conduct the patient to the anaesthetic room and the patient will be given an anaesthetic. When he or she comes round they will be in the recovery room, but they are unlikely to remember this. Most patients only remember waking up in their bed in the ward. Immediately after the operation the nurses will make frequent checks on the patient and will be ready to give the treatment ordered by the anaesthetist to reduce pain and nausea. Some patients will have a drip running into an arm vein so that they may have some fluid while they are unable to drink. The drip is removed when the patient feels better and starts to drink again.

Recovery after most cosmetic operations is really quite rapid and many patients are fit to go home (and rest) the next day. Post operative instructions should be followed as closely as possible because they are designed to prevent complications and ensure the best healing. Patients are usually given a telephone number to call in case of any problems and an outpatient appointment to see the surgeon in a few days. The immediate effect of a cosmetic operation tends to be swelling and bruising and the improvement in the appearance may take some time to become apparent.

THE CAUSES OF DISAPPOINTMENT

Although cosmetic surgery is generally very successful, even The Best Surgeon In The World occasionally has patients who are bitterly disappointed with their treatment. It may be because of problems in three main areas and these are sometimes combined.

The counselling stage – the surgeon and patient did not communicate properly so the patient didn't get the result he or she was expecting.

During the operation – perhaps a medical problem created a poor result. Or the standard of the surgery was simply not good enough. Surgeons are usually blamed if there are problems but there are many factors which can affect surgery which are not in the surgeon's control, however skilled and experienced he or she may be.

Afterwards – some sort of complication perhaps, or the patient is frustrated at the length of time it takes to recover or come to terms with the change in appearance.

COUNSELLING

Communication by talking is actually a very difficult skill and almost everyone occasionally misses the point or misunderstands when they talk to other people.

Spoken words conjure up images in the brain of the listener which can be totally different from those which were being described by the speaker. Words such as "small" or "better" can change their meaning entirely as they pass between the two. It is obvious that some surgeons, and of course some patients, are going to be better at communicating than others. Comfortable, stress-free conditions and enough time can make all the difference to the value of an interview. Many patients are nervous and embarrassed when they first meet a surgeon and these are barriers to effective communication. The surgeon should be able to relax the patient by a calm and unhurried approach. However good a surgeon is at operating he or she will never get the "Best Surgeon In The World" title if he or she does not make it easy for patients to talk about their problems.

If any patient after a consultation feels that they have not been able to say all they wanted to say, or felt that they were being misunderstood, they would be best advised to seek another consultation, possibly even see another surgeon, before they decide whether to have the operation.

At the initial consultation the surgeon will be carefully evaluating the patient's response to his questions and will be trying to decide exactly what the patient is hoping to get out of the operation. The result that the patient expects has to closely match the result that the surgeon is likely to achieve. If the patient is expecting something which is beyond the prowess of the surgeon, or is not a normal result of the operation itself, then disappointment is the likely outcome.

A few patients are disappointed with an operation which has been performed perfectly and where any objective observer would think there is an acceptable result. The problem here is that there has been a failure of communication between the patient and the surgeon. They both need to listen to each other. Photographs of the surgeon's previous patients are a great help because the patient can gain a good impression of what the operation can do for them and the surgeon can observe the patient's response. If these responses are inappropriate this is a warning sign to the surgeon. If the patient feels that the results shown in the photographs are disappointing because they fall short of what they are expecting then the patient must be warned that their expectations are probably unreasonably high and they must be advised not to proceed. If any patient forms the view in consultation with the surgeon that the surgeon's results will not please them then they would be foolish to go ahead.

Occasionally a patient changes his or her mind about the desired result during the course of the treatment. Whereas at the initial consultation they say that they are so bothered by their problem that they will accept any result, so long as it is an improvement, afterwards they are disappointed because the result is not perfect. The surgeon has done his best and come up with what the patient said would be acceptable but afterwards the patient has become more ambitious and then finds that a simple improvement is not enough.

The surgeon should be forthcoming about the negative side of the operation such as scarring or the possibility of the result changing with time. Any patient is likely to be disappointed if they did not know that an inevitable result of their operation is significant scarring for example. This is not always the fault of the surgeon; some patients simply do not listen when the operation is explained to them or they assume that in their case will be different or that the surgeon is trying to put them off for some reason.

All cosmetic surgeons occasionally see patients who they feel will not be happy afterwards. Some will plainly want an operation which either does not exist, or will not work in their case. Others will make the surgeon believe that however successful the operation is technically, it will not give them the result they want such as ensuring a major modelling contract or even attracting home an errant husband. Patient selection, that is only agreeing to operate on good candidates, is an important part of the surgeon's responsibility.

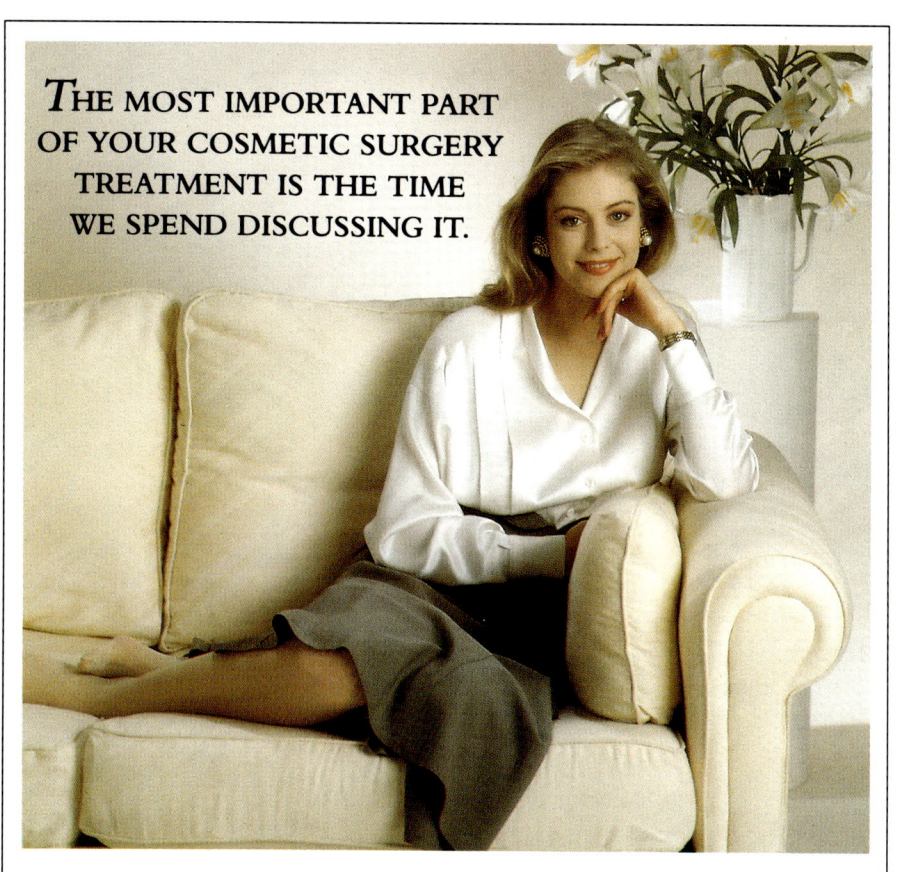

THE MOST IMPORTANT PART OF YOUR COSMETIC SURGERY TREATMENT IS THE TIME WE SPEND DISCUSSING IT.

Making a decision to undergo corrective cosmetic treatment is easier when you can discuss it with someone who is sympathetic, understanding and professional.

That's why, at the Harley Medical Group, the first thing we do is sit down and discuss exactly what we can do for you, the benefits, the actual procedures, and naturally the cost.

Should you decide – and there's no obligation – to proceed with treatment, we will go through each stage of the procedure in detail with you, tell you how long it will take and how much after care you will require.

Our range of corrective procedures includes body, breast, face, nose and ear-reshaping, eyelid surgery, Collagen replacement therapy, varicose and thread vein removal, permanent eyelash line enhancement, baldness reversal and a unique non-surgical treatment for the ageing face.

SKINCARE – Harley Medical Group skincare products now available from beauty salons and our clinics.

FOR A FREE CONSULTATION CALL YOUR NEAREST CLINIC

THE HARLEY MEDICAL GROUP

LONDON: 6 Harley Street, W1N 1AA. Phone 071-631 5494
MANCHESTER: 24a St John Street, M3 4DF. Phone 061-839 2527
BIRMINGHAM: 6 Chad Road, Edgbaston, B15 3EN. Phone 021-456 4334
BRIGHTON: 5 The Drive, Hove, East Sussex BN3 3JE. Phone 0273 324061

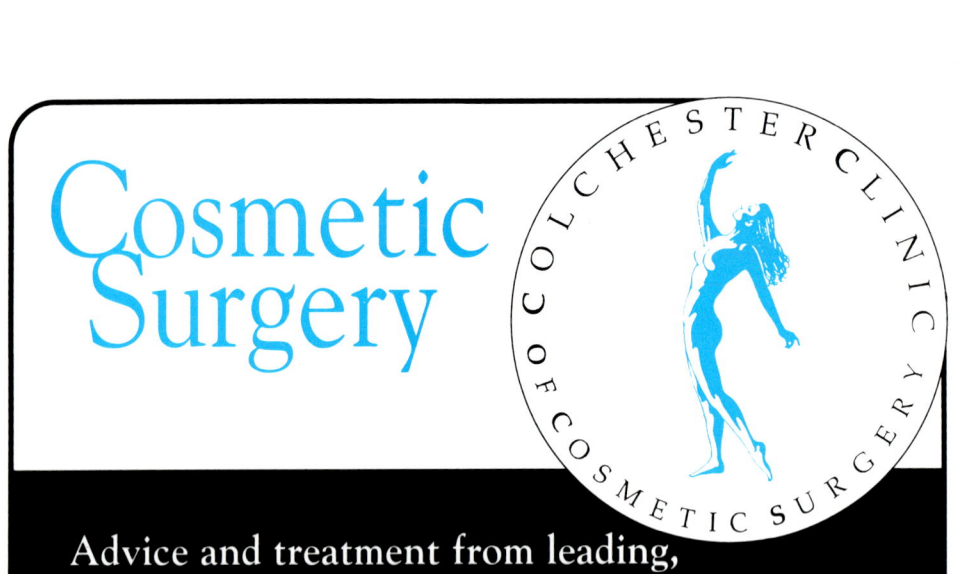

Cosmetic Surgery

COLCHESTER CLINIC OF COSMETIC SURGERY

Advice and treatment from leading, qualified cosmetic surgeons for men and women.

- Nose refinements & eye improvements
- Face lifts and spot fat reduction
- Bust enlargements
- Anti wrinkle treatments
- Collagen replacement therapy
- Varicose & thread vein therapy
- Micro hair grafts

For further details telephone:

(0206) 570980

**THE COLCHESTER CLINIC OF COSMETIC SURGERY
53 HEAD STREET, COLCHESTER, ESSEX, CO1 1NH**

DURING THE OPERATION

There is no substitute for skill and experience, and a genuine interest in cosmetic surgery, on the part of the surgeon. Every cosmetic surgeon is interested in how his patients look after the operation. Nevertheless all human beings occasionally make mistakes or errors of judgement and surgeons (and not just cosmetic surgeons) sometimes produce results which are not up to their usual standard. Sometimes this is a minor problem such as a misplaced suture slightly distorting the edge of a wound, or it could be a more significant error such as too much skin removed in trying to correct a crease. In general terms such consequences of surgery are unusual.

Much more likely is the situation where something happens which is outside the surgeon's control, such as an allergic drug reaction or where a patient has a bleeding tendency which was unsuspected before the operation. This can make the achievement of an optimum result very difficult indeed. Although technical perfection is the aim during the operation it is not always possible and the preoperative counselling of the patient should take this into account. Nowadays anaesthesia is not nearly as risky or a source of as many problems as it used to be and a healthy patient has little to fear from a routine anaesthetic.

AFTER THE OPERATION

A fully informed patient should be more relaxed after the operation and be better able to cope with minor discomfort and the appearance of the new wounds than someone who was unaware of the nature of the operation. Bruising, swelling and soreness are a feature of most operations and some patients complain that they were unprepared for this. They may also maintain that they did not realise that full recovery can take some time.

Post operative complications can occur as in all surgery. Especially important are the risks of infection and bleeding, both of which can mar an otherwise good result. Some areas of the body and some patients scar badly however neatly and expertly they are treated by the surgeon.

In general terms, if the result of a cosmetic operation is disappointing because of some technical problem it is nearly always possible by further revision surgery to correct the defect and produce a successful outcome.

In those unfortunate cases where there is a good technical result but where the patient is dissatisfied, further surgery is unlikely to be very effective and both surgeon and patient may come to regret the decision to operate.

ANAESTHESIA

Many patients are worried about having a general anaesthetic. Nowadays anaesthetics are rapid and safe. Once asleep the patient is in the hands of a trained specialist and is carefully watched during the entire procedure.

There are two types of anaesthetic, general and local. Under a general anaesthetic the patient is asleep but with a local anaesthetic only the part to be treated is made numb. Heavy sedation combined with local anaesthetic is called twilight sleep.

The type of anaesthetic which is used depends on the nature and extent of the operation and the wishes of the patient and surgeon. The patient's medical history or previous experience of anaesthetics can influence the decision.

GENERAL ANAESTHETIC

Before the operation Patients who smoke should give up or cut down as much as possible in the weeks before. It is also a good idea to drink less alcohol than usual especially in average or heavy drinkers. If a patient gets a cough or a cold or some other illness shortly before the date of admission he or she should inform the clinic because it might be sensible to postpone the operation.

If a patient is taking tablets or any medication he or she should bring them to the clinic. Some medical treatments can cause problems with anaesthetics. The anaesthetist will be particularly interested in previous anaesthetics that the patient has had and whether there was any trouble. Blood tests and urine tests may need to be done. Anaesthetics can make people sick. This can be dangerous so it is very important that the stomach is empty when the operation begins. Patients are not allowed to eat or drink for some hours before an operation. Sometimes a premedication, a sedative tablet or injection, is given about an hour before.

During the operation The patient is brought to the anaesthetic room which is usually a side room leading into the theatre. A careful check is made to ensure that no mistakes of identification have occurred and that the consent form for the operation has been signed. Often leads are attached to the body so that the heartbeat and breathing can be checked. One of the veins in the arm or hand is pricked with a small needle and the anaesthetist injects a drug which makes the patient rapidly go to sleep. Other drugs can be given to prolong the anaesthetic and often a tube is used to provide the patient with oxygen and anaesthetic gas during the procedure. Sometimes a drip, which is a thin plastic tube running from a bottle into a vein, is put up to give the patient some fluid, especially if the operation is going to take a long time.

At this point the patient is taken into the operating theatre and the operation begins. The anaesthetist keeps a very close watch on the patient and gives further drugs as necessary. When the operation has finished the patient is transferred to the recovery room an allowed to wake up. Often pain relievers and drugs to control nausea are given at this time. When the patient has recovered enough he or she is taken back to the ward and can then sleep off the rest of the anaesthetic.

After the operation Some patients will feel a bit groggy for a while, depending on the length of the operation, and often a bit sick. Nowadays recovery from a modern anaesthetic is much quicker than it used to be and the after-effects are much less severe. Strong drugs are available to deal with pain and feeling sick. It is the aim of the anaesthetist that the patient should remember the operation as being a pleasant experience.

If a patient leaves the clinic soon after the operation they may still be slightly under the influence of the anaesthetic and they must not drive or operate machinery until at least 24hrs after they have recovered.

Complications are rare after a routine general anaesthetic where there are no previous symptoms of ill health. There is however a small risk of chest infection, thrombosis in the veins of the legs and complications affecting the heart and circulation. Some patients may have allergic reactions to some of the drugs used and the anaesthetist will be ready to deal with any untoward events which occur.

LOCAL ANAESTHETIC

Some operations done under local anaesthetic are often very minor and the patient can be in and out of the clinic very quickly. In more major cases some or all of the procedures necessary for a general anaesthetic are employed. The patient generally remains awake during the operation, even if sedated. Recovery is very much quicker without the hangover-like after effects of a general anaesthetic. The anaesthetic is given by injecting it directly into the part which is going to have the operation. Within a very short time the area goes numb, an effect which can last for several hours. The post operative treatment depends on the nature of the surgery.

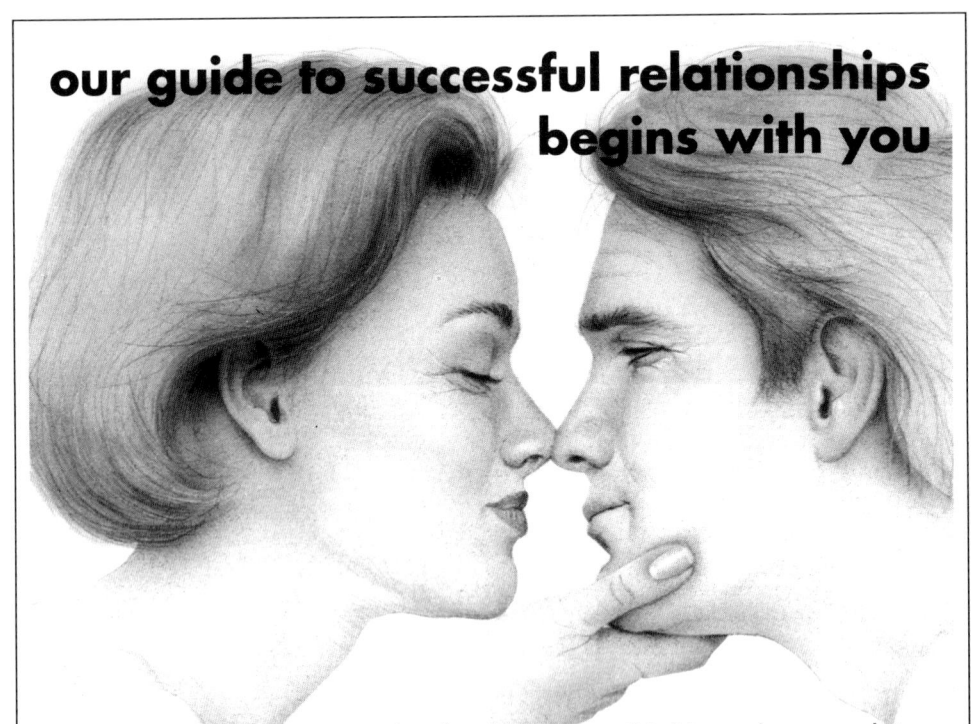

our guide to successful relationships begins with you

Feel confident about the way you look and we know that you'll feel better about your relationships. The Surgical Advisory Service has been helping people feel better about the way they look for almost a decade.

From the very first time you contact The Surgical Advisory Service you'll find you're in safe hands. Our fully-trained nurse-counsellor deals personally with every enquiry from the first time you get in touch, to your final discharge. Our surgeons are all members of The British Association of Cosmetic Surgery and Fellows of The Royal College of Surgeons.

Based at Marie Stopes House, in central London, we offer a complete range of facial and other cosmetic treatments which include: Face-lift; eyebag removal and eyelid rejuvenation; new non-surgical, fruit acid facial skin peel; liposuction and breast enhancement or reduction. Our minor surgery clinic offers collagen treatments to smooth away lines and wrinkles - the tell-tale signs of ageing; surgical procedures include vasectomy reversal; infertility treatments and male circumcision.

To arrange an initial consultation with our nurse-counsellor, or discuss how we can make it easier to pay for treatment, call direct on the numbers below, or write to us at Marie Stopes House.

071-388 1839 (tel)
071-383 5703 (fax)

THE SURGICAL ADVISORY SERVICE

Marie Stopes House
108 whitfield street london W1P 5RU
visa and access accepted

FACELIFT

This operation is so successful that the word facelift has now passed into general usage, meaning any procedure which produces a clear improvement in appearance. The purpose of a facelift operation is to raise and tighten the facial skin thereby eliminating or decreasing overhanging folds or lines. The standard facelift operation is effective in the neck, chin, cheeks and temporal regions, i.e. the lower two thirds of the face and neck. The forehead and eyelid regions are not included in the standard operation and require separate procedures which may be combined with it.

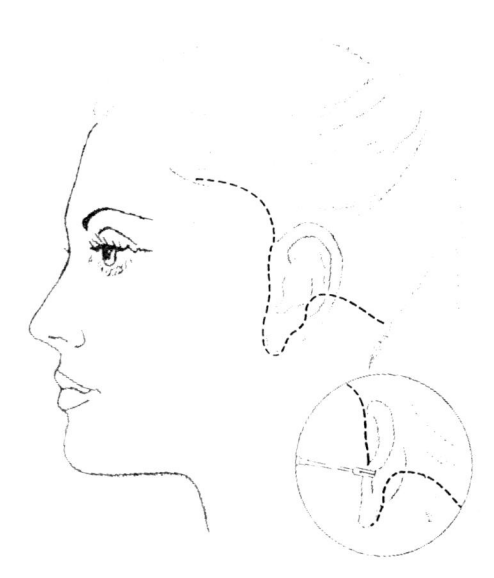

THE USUAL INCISION FOR A FACELIFT

It is not possible to eliminate every line, wrinkle or furrow in a facelift procedure. Prominent lines or wrinkles which remain will require additional treatment e.g. skin abrasion, collagen injections and fat implants. The improvement gained, that is the lessening of the signs of ageing compared to before the operation, is permanent. Sooner or later, the signs of ageing will return and this can sometimes be in as short a time as several months but is usually a number of years. If the patient wishes the operation can then be repeated to gain further benefit.

A general or twilight anaesthetic is usually administered. The incision begins in the temple behind the hairline and proceeds downwards in front of the ear. It then continues in the fold behind the ear and finally extends horizontally inside the hairline towards the back of the head. The skin is then gently lifted from the face and neck. The released skin is then stretched gently backwards and upwards and the excess is excised. The incisions are then sutured and the face is bandaged for 24 hours. The length of stay in hospital is generally no longer than two days and the sutures are removed at 5 to 10 days.

Afterwards there is often numbness, which usually resolves within a few weeks. There is always a change to the hairline in front of and behind the ear. This occurs because the facial skin has been moved to a new position. Bleeding sometimes occurs under the skin soon after the operation and may need treatment. Occasionally it can take a long time to heal behind the ear because of tension in the skin.

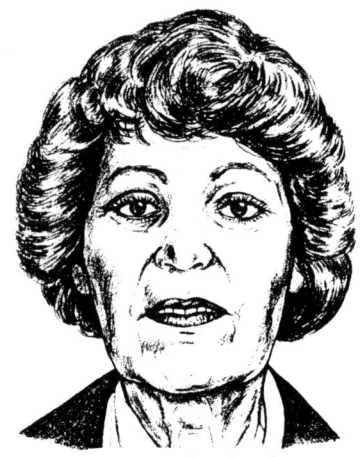

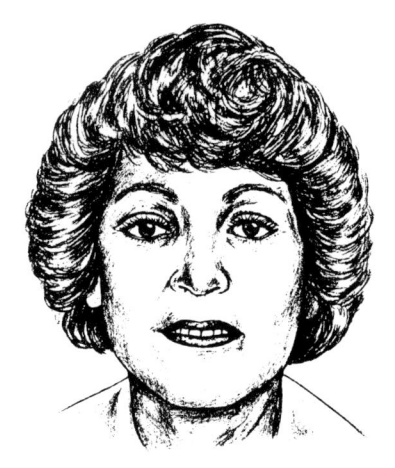

Patients who are good candidates for a facelift are likely to gain a very gratifying result. They can look years younger and this can be a great boost for their confidence, both in social situations and at work. The improvement in appearance can be dramatic and is usually even more so when combined with blepharoplasty (removal of eyebags) and dermabrasion to the upper lip.

Replace your skin's natural youthful suppleness instantly. You can take years off your appearance by losing wrinkles, creases and even skinfolds from around your eyes, nose and mouth.

JOHN BALLENTYNE
&
ASSOCIATES

Dental Surgeons
**24 Village Square,
Chelmer Village, Chelmsford
Telephone: (0245) 451324**

If you care about your looks consider collagen replacement therapy – it's the obvious choice!

KEEP YOUR YOUTHFUL APPEARANCE WITH COLLAGEN REPLACEMENT THERAPY

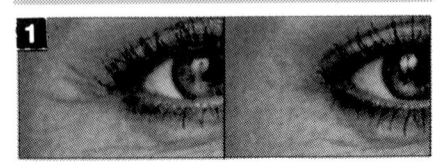

Lines around the eyes disappear. Creases around lips are removed with dramatic effect.

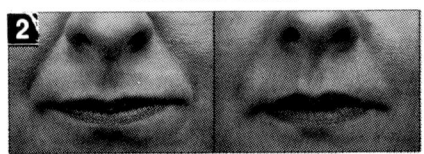

Call us now for a consultation and further details

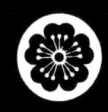

The HEATH CLINIC

offers the complete range of Cosmetic Surgery in a friendly, discreet and understanding atmosphere.

These services include:

- Breast enlargement & reduction
- Face lift & eyelid surgery
- Nose reshaping
- Chin, cheek & ear enhancement
- Abdominal reshaping
- Liposuction (fat removal)
- Varicose veins & thread veins
- Calf implants

For more information contact Marie Horan or Ciara Holland on

Telephone: 081-458 4416 or Fax: 081-905 5274

or write to:

**The Heath Clinic,
58 West Heath Drive, London NW11 7QH**

Licensed by Area Health Authority.
Recognised by major Medical Insurance Companies.

Please send me information on: (Please write in capital letters)

NAME _____

ADDRESS _____

_____

CS

THE
LIPS

With ageing the upper lip becomes less bulky with vertical crease lines. This is made much worse by smoking and also by losing the teeth. The creases are very effectively treated by dermabrasion or a deep chemical peel, which can be combined with a facelift. If the upper lip is long and the lips themselves are thin, a slip of skin can be removed from the lip margin which makes the lip pout more. This can also be done in young people. If the patient wants the lips to be more bulky, then either fat or collagen can be implanted along the lip margin. Collagen injections tend not to last for very long in this site.

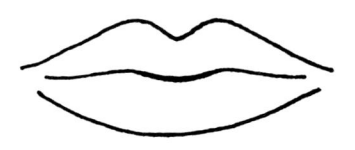

Oversized, thick lips can be reduced by taking out a slip of skin and underlying tissue from the inside. This operation is usually performed on Negros. Because the scars are inside the mouth they do not show and they are unlikely to form into unsightly lumps which can happen when Negros have scars on their skin surface. The swelling immediately after this operation can be quite dramatic but after a few weeks when the swelling has gone the lips will be much less fleshy. There is a limit to how much can be removed, because if too much is taken away the lips will not close properly.

EYELID SURGERY

With age the upper eyelid skin becomes stretched and slack and hangs as a fold over the eye. In the lower eyelid, fat from the eye socket pushes forward and creates a bulge. Treatment is aimed at reducing the amount of excess skin in the upper lid and reducing the bulge and tightening the skin in the lower.

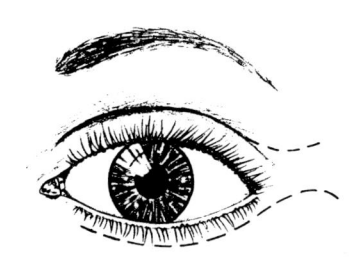

THE STANDARD INCISION FOR UPPER AND LOWER BLEPHAROPLASTY

The procedure is usually performed under sedation and local anaesthesia although a general anaesthetic is sometimes preferred for an exceptionally nervous patient. In the upper lid the incision is made in the lid crease. In the lower lid the incision starts at the outer side in a crow's foot and extends under the eyelashes. Through these incisions, excess fat, skin and if necessary muscle can be appropriately removed. Sutures are usually removed between three and five days.

Where there is just an eyebag and no spare skin on the lower eyelid it is possible to remove the eyebag, which is just a pad of fat by an approach from behind the eyelid. This technique has the advantage that it does not scar the skin. In many patients a supplementary technique such as a chemical peel is then used to remove any fine wrinkles still present on the lower eyelid.

Afterwards, swelling and bruising around the eyes is inevitable. The bruising usually subsides within ten days and scars can usually be camouflaged by makeup at that time. The eyes may be watery for a while. After several months the scars will fade and often become almost invisible. Minor degrees of swelling may persist for a few weeks afterwards. it is not possible to remove all creases from the lower lid. The skin often feels a little tight shortly after the operation. Eyelid surgery may cause the eyes to be rounder in shape than they were before. This is most likely to happen if a considerable amount of skin is removed. Contact lenses should not be worn for at least two weeks afterwards. Normal activities can be resumed in seven to fourteen days.

The result of a successful eyelid operation can be a dramatic improvement, extremely pleasing for the patient as well as long lasting. Eyelids without creases and bags will look much younger and the eyes often will look larger. it is often combined with a facelift.

CORRECTION OF THE ORIENTAL EYE

The essential difference between a Caucasian and Oriental upper eyelid is that the former has a transverse fold or crease above the eyelashes. It is possible to produce this fold with a surgical operation. This is very popular in some areas of the World.

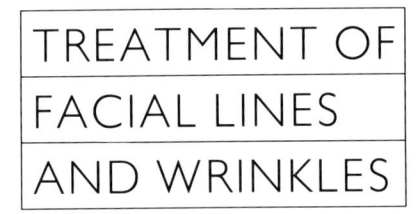

TREATMENT OF FACIAL LINES AND WRINKLES

Gradually our skin loses elasticity. Fine lines and wrinkles form as a consequence of the movements of facial expression and the effects of gravity. This process is accelerated by smoking and sunlight.

Wrinkles, scars and creases can be treated by one of two basic methods. Either they can be filled so that the depressions come up to the level of the highest parts, or the whole surface can be smoothed by reducing the highest parts to the same level as the lowest.

BACS
THE BRITISH ASSOCIATION OF COSMETIC SURGEONS

Surgery for the improvement of appearance has been undertaken by surgeons from many surgical disciplines. Ear, nose and throat surgeons were the first to carry out cosmetic rhinoplasty for example. Cosmetic surgery has been undertaken by general and orthopaedic surgeons, gynaecologists, opthalmic surgeons and many others long before plastic surgery became established as a separate speciality.

In recent years, plastic surgery which is a relatively new surgical speciality has tended to treat cosmetic surgery as part of its own broad speciality. This is very much against the history of cosmetic surgery which in the past has benefited from the multidisciplinary approach.

Some plastic surgeons have no interest in cosmetic surgery. They do not approve of it or carry it out. Most plastic surgeons perform cosmetic surgery privately in their spare time, outside the NHS, because cosmetic surgery is not readily available on the NHS.

In 1980 a small group of surgeons, some of whom were plastic surgeons and some from other disciplines, inaugurated the British Association of Cosmetic Surgeons. What united them was their interest in Cosmetic Surgery as a speciality in its own right.

The British Association of Cosmetic Surgeons was therefore established to promote the study and practice of Cosmetic Surgery and to act as a forum for the interchange of information and ideas among the members and to promote and maintain the highest standards of surgery.

The Association has grown over the years but has never lost sight of its initial aims. The entry criteria which have to be satisfied by new members are strict and membership is an honour. All members of the Association are Fellows of one or more of the Royal Colleges of Surgeons (FRCS) and have proven competence in Cosmetic Surgery. This requires years of study and practice after obtaining the Fellowship, usually under the supervision and tutorage of one of the senior members.

All members carry out Cosmetic Surgery as a major part of their practice or full time.

The Association holds regular meetings to discuss aspects of Cosmetic Surgery and many members travel widely abroad to attend meetings and conferences. Many recent advances in the field have been introduced to this country by members of the Association. Every member of the British Association of Cosmetic Surgeons is a trained cosmetic surgeon and has extensive experience in the speciality.

Further information on cosmetic surgery can be obtained from:
The British Association of Cosmetic Surgeons, 17 Harley Street, London W1N 1DA

Filling Materials

COLLAGEN

Collagen is a natural protein found throughout the body and is the main component of skin. Small depressions and creases in the skin can be injected with a small amount of highly purified animal collagen, which the body accepts as its own. It becomes a functioning part of the skin and even stimulates new natural collagen formation.

There are now several different types and strengths of collagen available. Each type is designed either for a specific area or for a particular kind of skin crease, wrinkle or fold. Before treatment can begin a small test dose is injected into the skin of the forearm as an allergy test. 97% of patients will show no reaction and can proceed with treatment. The result of the test is assessed after four weeks. Assuming there is no reaction, the treatment consists of a series of tiny injections into the wrinkles and is performed as an outpatient procedure.

Like the body's own collagen, the new collagen will gradually be depleted or absorbed by the body and further "top-ups" will be required every six to twelve months but this can be very variable. The amount of material used for these "top-ups" is much less than the original treatment but this will ensure that 100% correction of the defect is maintained.

Paris Lips Collagen implants as well as being used to fill out the small creases around the lips, can also be used to enhance the borders of the lips and give more definition. Younger patients may wish to have more prominent and "pouty" lips. This technique using collagen to produce this look has been named the "Paris Lip" after the French plastic surgeon who first created it.

SYNTHETIC INJECTABLE SUBSTANCES

Synthetic, non irritant, non absorbable substances which can be injected to fill out lines and wrinkles are being developed. The best known of which is microparticular silicone. This substance was developed to act as a permanent injectable filling agent which does not migrate. It is a suspension of tiny solid silicone particles suspended in an absorbable gel. These particles are unable to migrate beyond the site of injection. The material has a very thick consistency and can therefore only be injected through a large, blunt-ended needle. This makes its application limited to injections deep in the skin, such as nose, chin, cheeks, deep facial grooves and puckered scars. It is not suitable for the treatment of fine facial lines. The result is permanent, although it may be possible to remove the material surgically. It is common for the implanted area to become firm. This is not a problem if the material is used to augment a cheekbone for example but it does mean that microparticular silicone is not recommended to be used in the lips.

TRETINOIN

This is a derivative of vitamin A. Tretinoin increases the rate of skin cell turnover, increases the thickness of the skin and increases collagen deposition. The overall effect is that the skin becomes more youthful in appearance, with fine lines and wrinkles smoothed out. In addition tretinoin hastens the clearing of pigment-filled skin cells. As a result dark spots lighten and discolouration evens out. Tretinoin also helps eradicate precancerous skin changes such as actinic keratoses. It has been used by doctors for over 15 years and has proved to be a safe preparation. During the initial stages of application some patients may experience minor skin irritation, redness and burning sensation as well as peeling of the skin. Tretinoin increases the skin's sensitivity to ultraviolet radiation and prolonged exposure to the sun should be avoided.

Smoothing Procedures
DERMABRASION

Dermabrasion is a procedure used in selected cases to remove irregularities in the skin surface. A rotating wire brush or diamond wheel is used to plane down the irregular area. An improved appearance is obtained by making the surface uniform. Old acne scars and chicken pox marks can be improved as well as certain superficial skin discolourations. Dermabrasion is also used to treat fine lines and wrinkles especially those in the upper and lower lips. In severe acne scarring, several procedures will be necessary over a period of time. Small areas can be treated under local anaesthesia. Large areas are best treated under general anaesthesia. A scab develops on the abraded area within 1 or 2 days and gradually lifts off in 7 to 10 days depending on the depth of the abrasion. A smooth, pink skin results which gradually returns to normal colour in the next 6 to 8 weeks.

Pigment alteration occurs in all patients for several weeks. Initially the abraded area will appear pink and less pigmented than the surrounding skin. It may take up to 6 weeks to regain normal pigmentation. Final pigment adjustment may take several months. **It is important to remember that exposure to sunlight** within six or eight weeks following treatment **may result in brown or white blotchy discolouration.** All patients are strongly urged to stay out of the sun for this length of time and use emollient sunblock cream if exposed to sunlight. Dermabrasion and chemical peeling can be extremely difficult for a patient post operatively. Most patients would wish to stay out of the limelight until healing has occurred or until such time as make up can be applied to hide the initial effects.

The result of a successful dermabrasion can be a very dramatic improvement especially if the original blemish was very noticeable. Despite the horrendous initial appearance after the first 24 to 48 hours, patients cope very well.

CHEMICAL PEEL – CHEMABRASION

This procedure consists of applying strong chemicals (phenol, croton oil) which burn and remove the superficial layers of the skin in much the same way as occurs mechanically with dermabrasion. It is most commonly used for improving fine lines around the mouth and eyes, but large areas, even the whole face can be peeled under special conditions. The upper lip and brow are often treated in this way in conjunction with a facelift. Chemical peeling acts like dermabrasion by stimulating the patient's own collagen formation beneath the treated area. this rejuvenates the skin giving it a fresh, smooth appearance. It is very similar to dermabrasion in its post operative events. Crusting, tightness and redness will last for at least 10 to 14 days. Frequently pink discolouration will last three to four weeks. Although this is not a surgical procedure it can be painful for several days, particularly when the entire face is treated at one time. Temporary heart problems have occasionally been caused by the application of the chemicals. The procedure needs to be done where treatment for this problem is available. **Exposure to sunlight within six to eight weeks may result is discoloured patches.**

Both a deep facial peel or a dermabrasion can be dramatically successful in achieving a rejuvenation of the skin.

THE LONDON COSMETIC SURGERY CENTRE

Many people will admit to being concerned or unhappy about some aspect of their physical appearance. Medical advancement has not enabled many of these problems to be corrected or drastically improved safely and effectively with the minimum of inconvenience.

The London Cosmetic Surgery Centre refers patients directly to reputable full time cosmetic surgeons, bypassing non medically qualified "counsellors" or hard pressure sales persons thereby reducing the overall cost and providing the most ethical service possible.

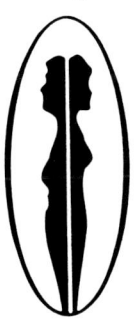

Some of the more popular procedures available include:

FACIAL REJUVENATION, Face Lift, Eyebag Removal, Brow Lift, Scar Revision, Dermabrasion, Collagen Replacement Therapy.

EAR & NOSE reshape.

BREAST ENLARGEMENT, Uplift, Reduction, Inverted Nipple Correction.

BODY CONTOUR SURGERY, Abdominal Reduction, Liposuction.

LIMBS, Liposuction, Varicose Veins, Spider Veins, Tattoo Removal.

The Clinic also specialises in the treatment of Male Pattern Baldness. All the latest treatments and technology are available.

For further information, please contact:
**THE LONDON COSMETIC SURGERY CENTRE
61 WIMPOLE STREET, LONDON W1M 7DE
TEL: 071-487 5736**

Consultations & Operations also available in Ireland, contact:
**THE DUBLIN COSMETIC SURGERY CLINIC
20 FITZWILLIAM PLACE, DUBLIN 2
TEL: DUBLIN 6611637, 6765650, 6762527**

CORRECTION OF PROTRUDING EARS

Otoplasty is an inherited condition where one or both of the ears may not grow into the normal shape. Surgery is often very helpful in improving the ears although sometimes it may not be possible to achieve an entirely normal appearance, especially in the worst cases. In adults it is often performed with a local anaesthetic.

Incisions are made in the groove behind the ear so that the scars are hidden from view. After the operation a bandage is usually applied for 24 hours. Thereafter a bandage is worn only at night for a few weeks.

Afterwards the ears will be swollen and bruised and they will be sore and tender for a day or two.

Sometimes the final position of the ears may prove to be unsatisfactory to the patient and a further procedure may be required. This is particularly so in cases of severe deformity. It is not reasonable to expect perfect symmetry because the two ears are never exactly alike, even in the normal state.

After the otoplasty the ears should look reasonably normal. This gives the freedom of choice to choose any hairstyle and avoids the difficulty of hiding them when going swimming or on windy days. This is one of the most frequent and successful operations in cosmetic surgery. The result is permanent and if performed early in life will prevent classroom teasing which can lead to serious psychological disturbances in the child and heartache to parents.

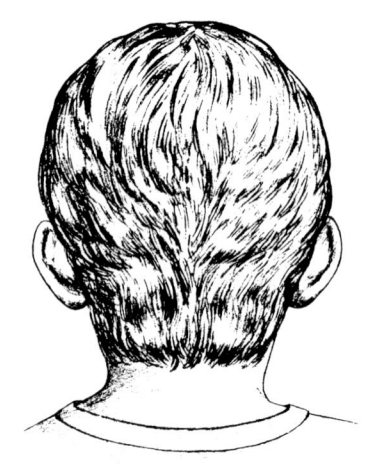

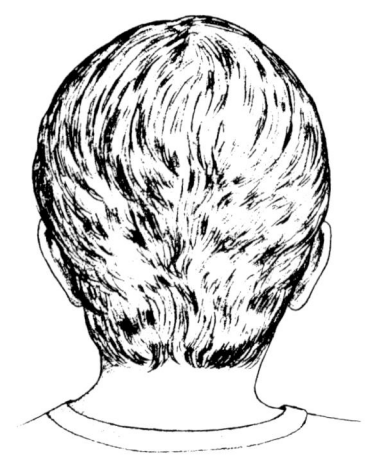

RESHAPING THE NOSE – RHINOPLASTY

Corrective nasal surgery is one of the commonest cosmetic pocedures performed today. The operation is performed for repair of injuries and also when the nose has become an ugly shape during growth.

Before the operation the shape of the new nose is carefully discussed. Pre-operative photographs are taken. The operation is usually done under general anaesthetic. The shape of the nose is changed along the lines agreed with the patient and is accomplished by removing, shifting or altering the underlying bony and cartilagenous structures. The skin then takes on the shape of the underlying frame. Generally the operation is performed from inside the nose leaving no external scars. Afterwards a plaster of Paris splint is placed on the nose and secured in position with sticky tape to the forehead and cheeks. This is removed after 10 to 14 days. The nose often looks rather pinched and thin when the plaster is removed.

Afterwards there will be bruising and swelling of the nose as well as around the eyes. Most of this subsides within a week, but slight swelling in the nose, which is not generally apparent to the onlooker, but which can be noticed by the patient, may take many weeks to subside. The thicker the skin covering the nose the longer it takes for the nose to attain its final shape. There is usually only very little pain. The nose can remain stuffy for some time after the operation and it is common for the tip to be numb for a while.

Most patients are delighted with the result of the operation which is generally very successful in improving the appearance of an ugly nose. However there is a limit to how much some noses can be changed. The surgical goal is improvement and it is not always possible to match the ideal which might be present in the mind of the patient. Noses which have been severely injured or those which are markedly crooked are technically difficult to correct and a second procedure may be necessary.

CHIN AUGMENTATION – MENTOPLASTY

Chin enlargement is performed either for a receding or weak chin or in conjunction with a nose reshape operation to achieve a better profile. A silicone chin implant (which is available from the manufacturers in various shapes and sizes) is inserted to lie against the front surface of the original chin via an incision inside the mouth. The operation therefore leaves no external scars.

Displacement of the implant can occur even if the implant was correctly inserted initially. Further surgery to put it back in the right place will be necessary.

Infection sometimes occurs and usually responds to antibiotic treatment. It can lead to extrusion of the implant. This will probably occur soon after the operation if it is going to but can sometimes happen many months afterwards. A further procedure will then be required to re-insert the implant at a later date.

Numbness of the lower lip often occurs. It is usually only temporary but on extremely rare occasions it can remain as a permanent feature.

The operation improves the shape of the chin and the balance of the face. This will be permanent once the wound around the implant has fully healed.

Implants can also be placed on the underside of the chin to make the lower part of the face longer, but they are not very stable unless secured into position in some way and this makes the operation more complicated. They are inserted through an incision in the skin just below the jaw in the midline.

If the jaw is too long, then a small amount of bone can be removed from the point of the jaw, either from the front or underneath. Unfortunately the roots of the teeth and the shape of the jaw itself often limit the amount of bone which can be removed, and therefore only fairly minor changes can be achieved by this method. The incision is made on the underside of the jaw in the natural crease and if there is any redundant skin as a result of the bone removal then it can be easily excised leaving a single scarline.

Occasionally patients request that various alterations are made to the actual shape of the chin, such as producing a cleft or making a dimple. It is possible to do this in some cases.

CELLULITE REMOVAL

The world's first medically proven treatment for cellulite.

Most women suffer from cellulite – the unsightly dimpled orange peel effect on thighs, buttocks and tummy. It is notoriously difficult to dispel being resistant to conventional diets and exercise.

But now, a new non-surgical medical treatment, Cellulolipolysis, already benefiting 50,000 women in Continental Europe, is available in the UK from The Harley Medical Group. Recent clinical trials at a London teaching hospital have conclusively proved its effectiveness.

6 one hour treatments under medical supervision are all you will need. The result is smoother skin, a usual reduction of 1 to 2 clothes sizes in areas treated and long lasting relief from this embarrassing problem.

FOR A CONSULTATION WITHOUT CHARGE PLEASE TELEPHONE:

LONDON:	071-631 5494
MANCHESTER:	061-839 2527
BIRMINGHAM:	021-456 4334
BRIGHTON:	0273 324061

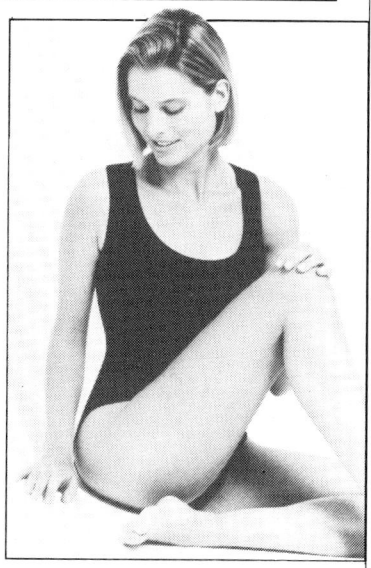

THE HARLEY MEDICAL GROUP
6 Harley Street, London W1N 1AA

Our corrective procedures for women and men include body, breast, face, nose and ear re-shaping, eyelid surgery, Collagen replacement therapy, skincare programme, varicose and thread vein removal, permanent eyelash line enhancement, baldness reversal and a unique non-surgical treatment for the ageing face.

BREAST AUGMENTATION (ENLARGEMENT)

Breast enlargement is one of the commonest cosmetic procedures performed. Approximately two million American women have had breast implants, either for reconstruction after breast cancer surgery or to enlarge or reshape the breasts. Most of these women have not experieced any serious adverse effects. But like all medical procedures, breast implantation does pose some risks and a woman must decide if she is willing to accept these risks in order to achieve the expected improvement in her appearance.

In general two groups of women seek breast enlargement. The first group consists of those who have never had a full development of breast tissue. The second group consist of those who have had normal breast development but whose breasts have decreased in size following pregnancy, increasing age or loss of weight.

Unfortunately there are no exercises or medications which can safely, effectively and permanently increase breast size. The only recognized and accepted method involves the insertion of a silicone breast implant behind the beast tissue.

A general anaesthetic is used in most cases. The site of the incision (usually about 3–4cms in length) will be chosen by the surgeon. It is generally made in the crease underneath the breast. Some surgeons however prefer to make the incision in the armpit or around the areola. A pocket for the implant is then made behind the breast, and a silicone implant is then inserted. The implant may be placed either in front of or behind the muscle of the chest. The implants come in different sizes and the surgeon will choose one which is most suitable.

On rare occasions after the operation bleeding may occur into the pocket created for the implant resulting in a haematoma. If a significant amount of blood collects, it may have to be removed, necessitating a further procedure.

Infection is unusual after this operation but may lead to the breakdown of the

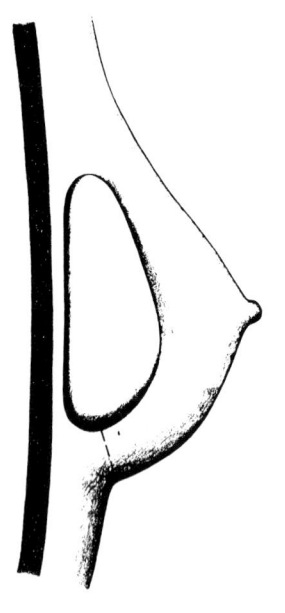

USUAL LOCATION OF SILICONE BREAST IMPLANT

incision necessitating the temporary removal of the implant. It usually occurs if it is going to, within the first ten days after the operation. After the infection has subsided the implant can safely be reinserted.

Whenever any foreign material is implanted, the body forms a protective shell of fibrous tissue called a capsule around the implant. The majority of these capsules are soft and yielding, so that in the case of a breast implant they will not alter the shape or the consistency of the breast. Unfortunately in some cases, after some time the capsule may shrink around the implant, compressing it and making it feel hard. Only a few capsules cause problems and in these cases the patient becomes aware of firmness and sometimes the breast changes shape. There may also be some discomfort. The manufacturers of implants have made improvements to the design recently which has reduced the incidence of these problems. If hardening does occur the breasts can be manipulated by the surgeon in a manner which breaks up the capsule thereby rendering the breast soft again. The problem can still recur. Only rarely is further surgery necessary.

Nearly every woman has breasts which are obviously asymmetrical at first glance and the breat augmentation operation does not normally correct this. Displacement of the implants can occur which can make this asymmetry worse. This can occasionally happen as a result of manipulation to soften them. The implant would then need to be repositioned by a second procedure. Occasionally a breast can become misshapen if the capsule becomes very thick or contracts excessively.

Some impairment of sensation in the nipple area may occur following surgery. Usually the sensation returns to normal in a few weeks. Very rarely is sensory loss a permanent feature. Sometimes the nipple area can become extra sensitive temporarily. In addition sensation in the lower portion of the breast may be impaired until the sensory nerves have recovered. Some patients report temporary "electric shock" type sensations lasting for a few moments. These mostly settle in time.

Modern implants are extremely difficult to burst or rupture. It is possible, but unlikely, for an implant to burst as a result of a severe blow on the chest such as in a car crash. Very occasionally an implant may rupture during manipulation of the breast when attempting to break down a capsule. if a ruptured implant is suspected it can be diagnosed by a mammogram.

Concern has been raised in the media about the possibility that leakage of silicone from breast implants can cause health problems. Actually the amount of silicone that leaks through the shell of modern implants is microscopic and no health problems have ever been shown to be associated with this. It is actually quite difficult to avoid silicone in ordinary life as it is a common constituent of food packaging and is found in many cleaning agents. It is very widely used in medicine in silicone tubing, artificial joints, cardiac pacemakers and the lubrication of hypodermic needles. Even over-the-counter indigestion remedies contain silicone which is absorbed by the stomach. No documented health hazards have ever been proven to have resulted from the presence of small quantities of silicone in the body.

Extensive research has been carried out to make sure that breast implants do not increase the risk of breast cancer. The results of this research show that there is no evidence that breast implants increase the chance of future development of cancer of the breast. If a lump appears in the breast after the operation, because all the breast tissue is in front of the implant, there should be no difficulty in detecting the lump and treating it if necessary. There is no doubt that the presence of breast implants can affect the ability of a radiologist to interpret mammograms (breast X-rays) and could hinder the detection of early cancer by this method. There are now techniques which overcome this problem and research has shown that mammograms are just as useful in detecting early breast cancer in those with implants as in those without.

There have been published reports which have suggested that silicone is implicated as a cause of autoimmune diseases but further research has shown that this suggestion is quite unjustified and there is no evidence that silicone is a cause of arthritis or any other serious health problem.

The implants do not interfere with breast feeding.

Implants show up on X-rays and therefore will be spotted by the radiologist. There is an old myth that implants may burst at high altitude in aircraft. This is quite untrue. There is also no evidence that modern implants degrade with time or wear out in any way and therefore they should certainly last the lifetime of the patient.

Breasts which were droopy before the operation will droop more after the insertion of implants unless a properly fitted support bra is worn.

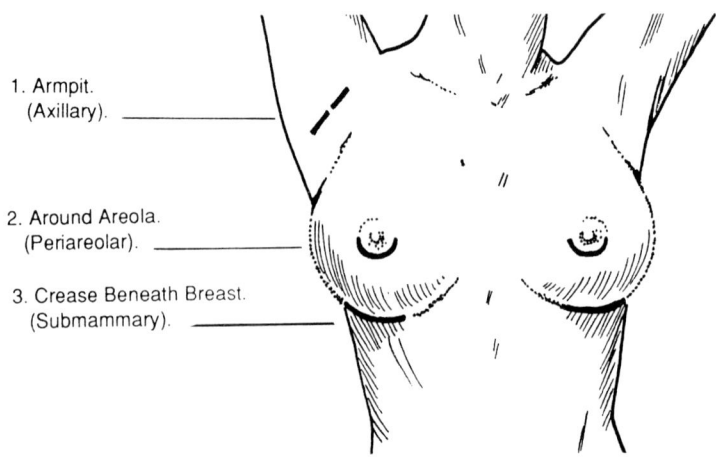

1. Armpit. (Axillary).
2. Around Areola. (Periareolar).
3. Crease Beneath Breast. (Submammary).

INCISIONS USED IN BREAST AUGMENTATION

Breast augmentation boosts the self confidence of women who would otherwise feel inadequate in certain clothes, on the beach and in sexual relationships. Research has shown that there is a significant psychological benefit in that over 90% of patients have increased self esteem and feeling of self worth following the operation, due to a more balanced perception of their body image. Most patients are completely comfortable with the change to their breasts and cease to be aware of the implants after a few weeks. With modern technology the newer breast implants now available have markedly reduced the incidence of hardening which is the one major problem which could mar an otherwise perfect result.

FOR INFORMATION, HELP & ADVICE
AND THE ARRANGEMENT OF CONFIDENTIAL
CONSULTATION ON ALL ASPECTS OF COSMETIC,
RECONSTRUCTIVE AND PLASTIC SURGERY CONTACT:

THE CAMBRIDGE CENTRE FOR COSMETIC SURGERY

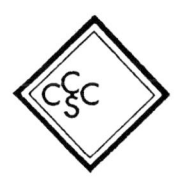

**FOR FREE BROCHURE
RING OR WRITE
CAMBRIDGE
(0223) 208085**

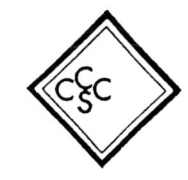

9.30 am–1 pm 2 pm–5.30 pm 24 hour message

**THE GRANGE, CAMBRIDGE ROAD,
NEW WIMPOLE, CAMBRIDGE SG8 5QD**

BREAST UPLIFT – MASTOPEXY

This operation lifts saggy breasts but does not change the size. A droopy breast can be restored to a much more youthful shape. It is also used to improve breasts which can have an unusual form. A mastopexy can produce a more normal appearance by lifting the nipples to a better position and changing the position of the crease underneath.

The most common reason for having the operation is where the breasts are droopy with the nipples lying lower than the breast crease. If the nipple is above the crease then the breast augmentation is a better operation. After having children, often the skin of the breast is stretched and the contents of the breast have shrunk so that the skin no longer fits nicely around the breast tissue. The aim of the operation is to reduce the amount of skin and lift the nipple.

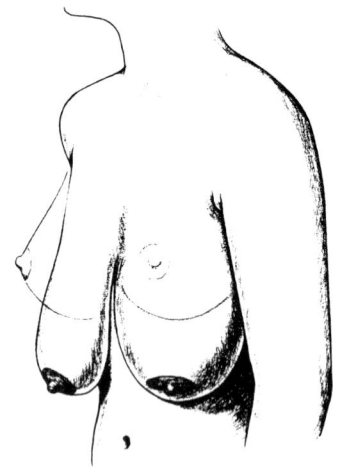

If the breasts are droopy simply because they are very big then a breast reduction should be performed. if, on the other hand, the breasts are still going to be too small even if they are raised to a better position, then mastopexy can be combined with augmentation. There are no exercises which are capable of shrinking stretched skin. Once the breasts have become saggy exercises will not help. A good supporting bra, worn routinely (especially during pregnancy) is the best prevention.

Before the operation the new site for the nipple is marked with a patient standing. Under general anaesthetic an incision is made around the edge of the areola and a lot of skin on the lower part of the breast is removed, but not the breast tissue. The nipple is lifted to its new position, often a few inches higher, and the skin is brought together underneath. After the wound is sutured a padded dressing is applied and the patient goes home the following day.

The main problem with this operation is the scarring. The surgeon will try to make the wound look as neat as possible, but it is unlikely that the scar will ever completely disappear. They may even stretch or become red and raised and require further treatment. Usually there is a scar around the areola, then a vertical part

BODY IMPROVEMENTS

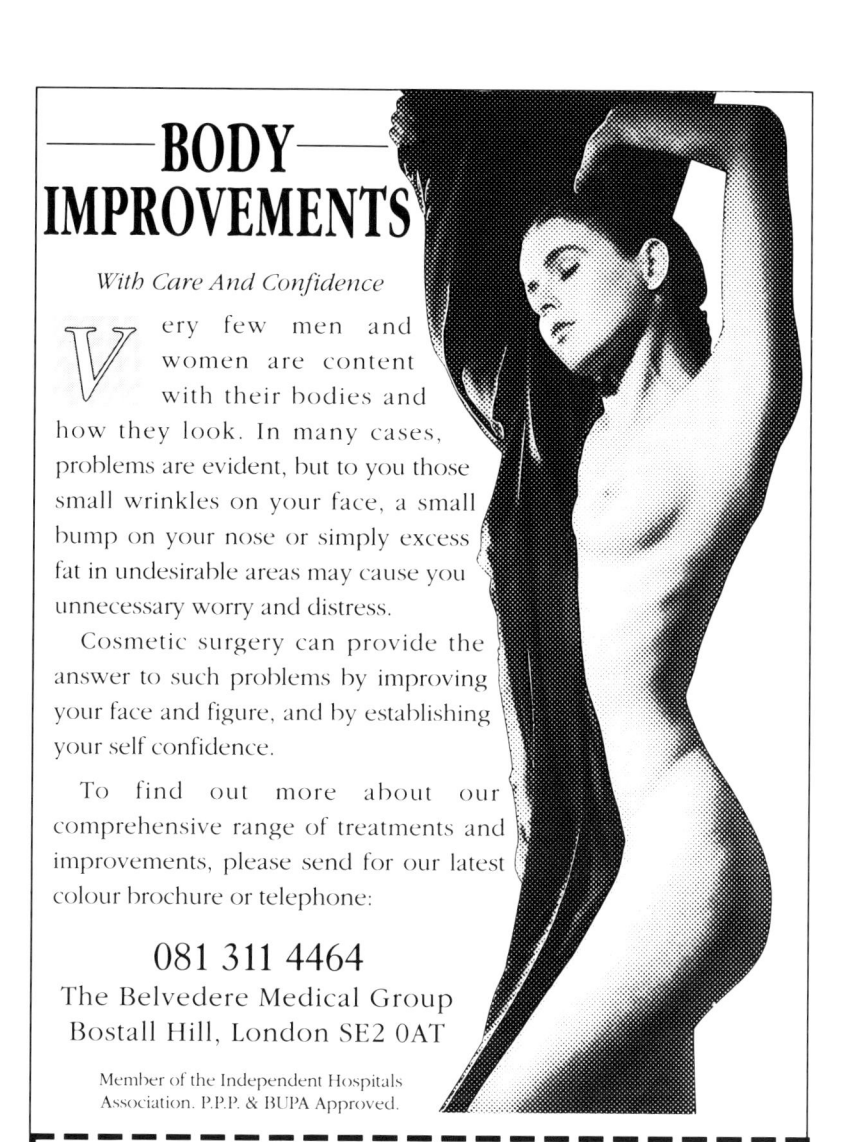

With Care And Confidence

Very few men and women are content with their bodies and how they look. In many cases, problems are evident, but to you those small wrinkles on your face, a small bump on your nose or simply excess fat in undesirable areas may cause you unnecessary worry and distress.

Cosmetic surgery can provide the answer to such problems by improving your face and figure, and by establishing your self confidence.

To find out more about our comprehensive range of treatments and improvements, please send for our latest colour brochure or telephone:

081 311 4464
The Belvedere Medical Group
Bostall Hill, London SE2 0AT

Member of the Independent Hospitals Association. P.P.P. & BUPA Approved.

The Belvedere Medical Group Bostall Hill, London SE2 0AT

Please send me your brochure ❏ Type of treatment(s) ....

NAME .... (C.S.G.)

ADDRESS ....

....

POSTCODE .... TELEPHONE ....

from the the edge of the areola going downwards and a variable length scar in the crease underneath.

In some patients there is a risk that the problem can recur, that is the breasts might become droopy again afterwards. The chance of this happening is reduced by wearing a well-fitting support bra afterwards. The sensitivity of the nipples may be reduced or altered although in all but a tiny minority this will return to normal.

In carefully selected patients and with optimum healing of the scars the results of mastopexy are very pleasing. The operation is not recommended for the young woman who is likely to have more children. If a patient does get pregnant afterwards the operation does not affect breast feeding.

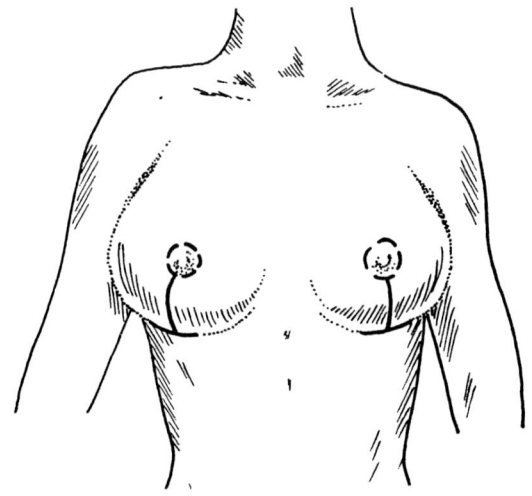

POSITION OF SCARRING IN MASTOPEXY

Northern Clinic of Cosmetic Surgery Health & Beauty

VISIT US WITH YOUR WRINKLES...

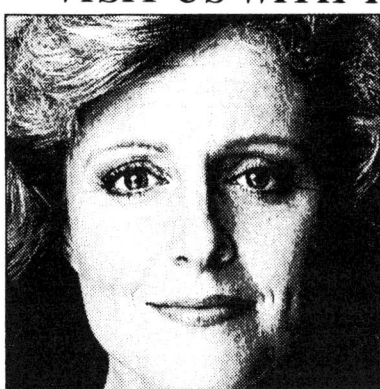

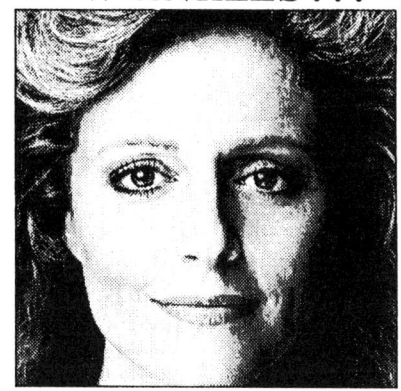

...AND LEAVE WITHOUT THEM!

"These improvements are achieved by Collagen Replacement Therapy"

We also specialise in the full range of cosmetic surgery techniques including face/neck lifts, upper/lower eye bag removal. Nose, ear and chin re-shaping. Breast enlargement/ reduction and uplift. Tummy tucks, varicose vein removal as well as liposuction i.e. spot fat reduction to areas that will not respond to diet and exercise (including male breasts), as well as the treatment of thread veins.

For your FREE consultation call

PRESTON (0772) 880032

16 WINCKLEY SQUARE, PRESTON PR1 3JJ
Also at: The Newlands Medical Centre, Bolton

BREAST REDUCTION

Large breasts can be a source of major embarrassment. As well as the difficulty of finding clothes that fit and look elegant, they tend to interfere with active sports. Sometimes they also cause backache and their weight makes the bra straps dig in over the shoulders. There is a tendency towards skin problems in the crease below each breast. With the passage of time they will hang lower and lower and the skin can become stretchmarked. Reducing the size of the breasts is a major operation.

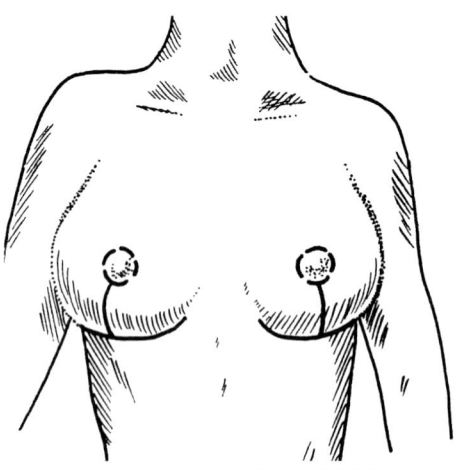

POSITION OF SCARRING IN BREAST REDUCTION

Several different techniques are used but they all cause quite significant scarring. The most usual method leaves a scar which runs around the edge of the areola and one in the crease underneath the breast and a vertical scar linking the two. These scars do not usually show outside an ordinary bra or bikini top. Although in most patients they fade with time they should be considered to be permanent.

Before the operation the new site of the nipple is marked on each side; it is often a few inches above the original position. Under general anaesthetic an incision is made around each nipple and a shape is cut in the skin to allow the skin and breast tissue to come together again after the redundant breast tissue and skin have been removed. The nipple is inset into its new site and the remaining breast tissue and skin are brought together beneath it. In very large breasts sometimes the nipple is taken off completely and placed in its new site as a skin graft. Normally the nipple is carried on bridges of skin to its new position which helps it retain a blood and nerve supply. The skin is sutured usually with absorbable sutures and a padded dressing is applied. Most patients are fit enough to go home two days afterwards.

Partial or even total loss of the nipple or areola can occur. If this happens it will need to be reconstructed. The sensitivity of the nipples may well be reduced or altered.

The scars may stretch and become red and raised. If the scars do not heal well they can generally be improved about a year after the original operation. Every attempt is made to make the scars as neat and inconspicuous as possible but they will always show on close examiantion. The shape of the breasts may look quite odd initially but as time passes they will settle down to look more natural. It is unlikely that the breasts will have a perfect shape or be exactly symmetrical.

Breast feeding is not usually possible afterwards and indeed it is very important that pregnancy is avoided for several years because the scars will stretch badly during pregnancy unless they are completely mature.

Some surgeons have described this operation as one of the most gratifying in the whole of surgery with an extremely high success rate despite the extensive scarring. Patients say that it is like an enormous weight has been lifted. They can go on the beach without embarrassment and fit into ordinary clothes. After the operation most patients feel a tremendous sense of freedom because they can do all the things that their large breasts stopped them doing before.

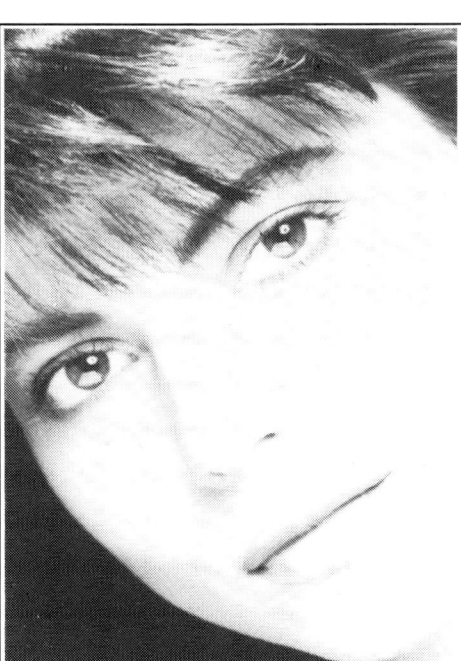

THE LOOKS YOU ALWAYS DESIRED

We believe that no-one need feel unhappy about their appearance. For years we have helped thousands of women and men to attain their dreams.

Recent advances in surgical skills mean that cosmetic surgery can be carried out with minimum inconvenience, often without needing a hospital stay.

We offer an outstanding blend of experience and reliability.

- TOP PLASTIC SURGEONS
- THE VERY LATEST TECHNIQUES
- A TOTAL FULLY INCLUSIVE FEE

Also a complete range of non surgical skin treatments and permanent hair transplanting. FREE Consultation.

For a FREE exploration of your individual needs meet our expert counsellor or use our professionally manned helpline anytime

THE AESTHETIC
PLASTIC SURGERY
ADVISORY SERVICE

NATIONAL HELPLINE
021 643 7515
Open 7 days a week 9.00am to 9.00pm

BIRMINGHAM, 150 NEW STREET, B2 4PA. LONDON, HARLEY STREET, W1.
MANCHESTER, ST JOHN STREET, M3 4DW. LEEDS, DUNCAN STREET, LS1 6DL.
LIVERPOOL, 45 RODNEY STREET, L1. BELFAST, 62A BLOOMFIELD AVENUE, BT5.
Also at Madrid, Lisbon and Rio.

GYNAECOMASTIA – MALE BREAST REDUCTION

Gynaecomastia is an enlargement of the male breast as a result of an abnormal increase in the glandular (breast) tissue. During adolescence it is common for the male breast to enlarge and later to decrease to normal size before the age of 21. Breast enlargement in an adult male may be due to excess fatty tissue or a combination of fatty and glandular tissue. Gynaecomastia in the late adolescent and adult male may be associated with hormone disorders, hormone producing tumours, liver disease and other rare abnormalities. In addition various drugs if taken for long enough can give rise to this embarrassing condition. Usually though, no underlying cause is found.

Patients seek treatment because of the embarrassment they suffer. In some patients pain and discomfort are additional problems. Before surgery is considered each patient must be fully tested to exclude any sinister cause for this condition.

General anaesthetic is usually employed. These days the operation is usually performed by using the technique of liposuction, with sometimes direct excision of the glandular tissue. Tiny incisions are made at the periphery of the areola and at other sites on the chest (depending on the surgeon's preference) for the introduction of a blunt metal tube to suck out the fatty tissue. Glandular tissue cannot be treated in this way and requires excision through an incision near the areola. Patients are usually fit to be discharged home the next day and sutures are removed at 7 to 10 days. Pressure dressings if used are left on for 7 days and many surgeons advocate the patient wearing an elasticated garment for several weeks afterwards. Normal exercise can be resumed as soon as the patient feels comfortable.

It is not possible to guarantee perfect symmetry of the breasts as most breasts are asymmetrical to begin with. occasionally the breast contour may be irregular and ruts and depressions can occur requiring further surgery.

Removing a significant volume of breast tissue beneath the skin in this situation can result in loose skin. The skin will recoil to a certain extent depending on the individual, but if it remains unsightly a further procedure can be performed to tighten it. This would result in noticeable scarring.

Nipple, areola and skin loss can occur as a result of poor circulation to these areas after the operation. Fortunately this complication is rare.

The result of the operation is permanent and should free the patient from embarrassment on the beach or in other situations where clothes cannot hide the abnormal breast development.

A skin problem is now something you can disguise.

If you suffer from skin problems like port wine birthmarks, scarring, severe acne or other disfiguring conditions, our camouflage service could be very good news.

We provide special camouflage creams and our make-up artist will teach you how to apply these to make the most of your looks.

Everyone has the right to look good and our make-up experts, as a vital part of one of London's finest Plastic and Reconstructive Surgery Units, are the best people to help you.

For more information on our Camouflage Advice and Make-up Service, or for an appointment, please call 071-586 5959 and ask for the Plastic and Reconstructive Surgery Unit.

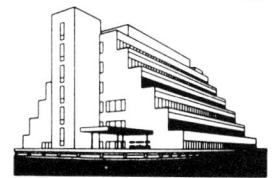

The Wellington Hospital
WELLINGTON PLACE, LONDON NW8 9LE.

CORRECTION OF INVERTED NIPPLES

In the majority of cases inverted nipples occur as a result of a defect in their development. Women who used to have normally protruding nipples but who find that they have become inverted later on in life should be fully investigated to exclude the possibility of underlying breast disease, most importantly cancer, which occurs in one in fourteen women in Great Britan.

Surgery to correct inverted nipples can usually be performed under local anaesthetic as a day case. Occasionally an overnight stay in a clinic may be recommended. Generally a small incision is made near the base of the nipple. Several different techniques can be used depending on the exact nature of the abnormality and the preferences of the surgeon and patient. Sutures may be removed after one week.

Afterwards breast feeding may prove difficult or impossible due to the fact that the milk ducts in the nipple are often affected by the operation.

The sensation to the nipple may be permanently impaired or even lost after surgery. Usually some loss of sensation is experienced by most patients which gradually returns to normal in time.

It is still possible for the nipples to invert again after the operation, even after the most expert surgery and a further correction may be required.

The usual result is entirely normal-looking nipples which react normally to temperature changes and being touched.

Guy's Nuffield House

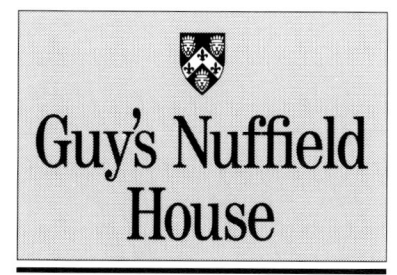

Cosmetic Surgery

Guy's Nuffield House part of the internationally known Guy's Hospital in central London now offer a full range of cosmetic surgery procedures to private patients.

For those seeking confidential professional advice and treatment at the highest level, 24 hour specialist care and superb facilities, Guy's Nuffield House should be your choice for cosmetic surgery procedures.

The income generated from Guy's Nuffield House is invested in Guy's Hospital for the benefit of its patients.

For confidential information, without obligation, please telephone:

071 955 4759/4760

Guy's Nuffield House, Newcomen Street, London SE1 1YR

BODY CONTOUR SURGERY – LIPOSUCTION

Liposuction (fat suction) has revolutionized body contour surgery in recent years and is now an approved and accepted method of removing specific areas of unwanted fat. Liposuction is not a method of reducing weight in the obese patient. It is a technique designed to resculpture nearly all parts of the body which have stubbon areas of fat that do not respond to diet or exercise. Liposuction can benefit many patients where previous techniques of body contouring were inadequate in achieving the desired result. It can also be combined with other standard procedures thereby producing better and longer lasting results such as in facelifting or abdominal lipectomy.

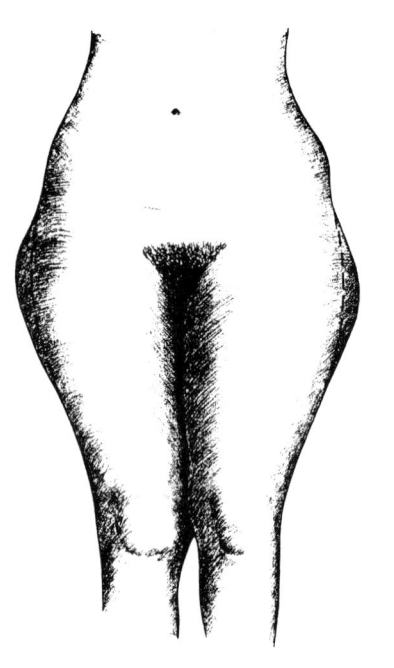

RESULT WITH LIPOSUCTION

The procedure is usually done under a general anaesthetic. A number of small incisions are made to allow a metal tube to be passed into the area of the unwanted fat. The fat is removed by powerful suction until a satisfactory shape is achieved. The length of the stay in the clinic is usually no longer than 2 days. The scars are usually tiny and are placed in sites which are not easily conspicuous. Most surgeons recommend that patients were an elasticated garment over the treated area constantly for several weeks. There is a wide variety of liposuction garments now available for all areas of the body.

Rippling and sagging of the skin can occur if either too much fat is removed from an area or if the skin is of such a poor tone initially that removing even a small amount of fat will exacerbate this effect. As a general guide, those patients who are under the age of 35 years old have a much better chance of a satisfactory result. It may be impossible to predict accurately how much the skin will recoil and take up the slack after the operation. Some patients will not accept loose skin in return for a more pleasing contour whereas others will do so quite happily.

Ruts and depressions in the skin can occur as a result of too much fat having been removed from a particular area. Although this complication can occur with any operator it is much less common in experienced hands. A further procedure may be required to improve the situation.

It is not possible to promise the patient perfect symmetry after the operation as the body is often asymmetrical to begin with. Where an obvious asymmetry results, further surgery may be necessary to correct it.

Changes in sensation can occur in the treated area due to minor nerve damage and may take some time to resolve completely. Various sensations have been described by patients such as stiffness, pins and needles, sensations like electric shocks and persistent discomfort. Usually however these symptoms settle in time.

Liposuction is an extremely successful operation permanently removing unwanted pads of unsightly fat. As with any other cosmetic operation this can bring increased confidence and happiness to the patient.

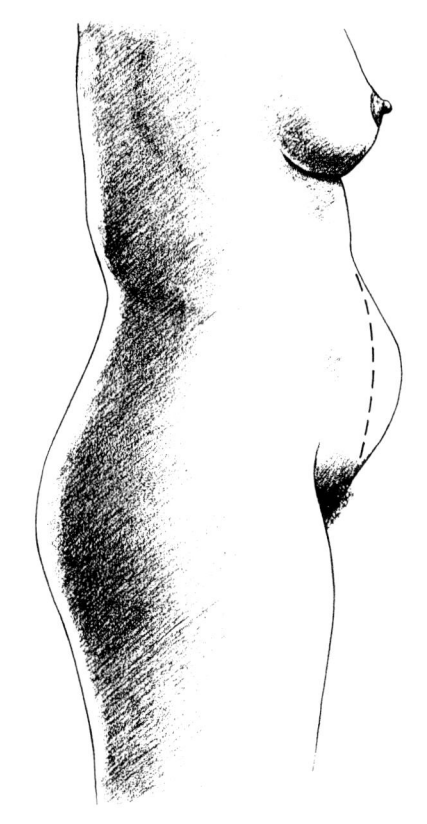

RESULT WITH LIPOSUCTION

ABDOMINAL LIPECTOMY – TUMMY TUCK

The tummy tuck removes excess skin and fat from the abdomen. The surgeon can tighten the tummy muscles at the same time. Most surgeons add liposuction to the standard procedure as it improves the result in suitable cases. The usual candidates are patients whose abdomens have stretched and sagged after losing weight or having children. This operation will not remove large amounts of weight from the obese patient. In fact there will usually be hardly any weight loss as a result of the operation. Apart from improving the profile, the procedure helps to remove stretch marks and scars from the lower part of the abdomen. Patients who have lost massive amounts of weight often have an apron of skin hanging down. They can get chafing and rashes under this apron and these are difficult to control. Also it is difficult to find clothes that fit and those which do are not flattering.

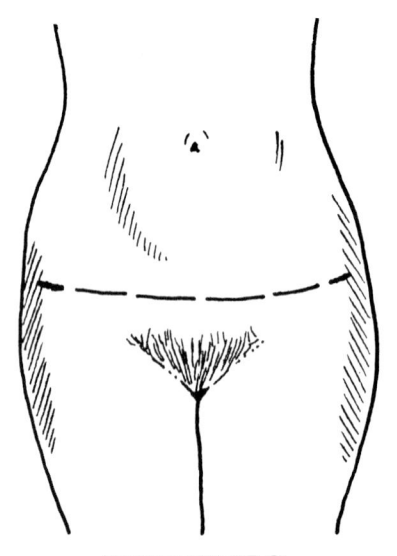

STANDARD TUMMY TUCK (ABDOMINOPHLASTY) INCISION. THE POSITION AND SHAPE CAN VARY ACCORDING TO THE INDIVIDUAL PROBLEM AND THE SURGEON'S PREFERENCE

A general anaesthetic is necessary. Fat is sucked away from the abdomen as necessary. The operation starts with a horizontal incision in the so-called "bikini line". The surgeon then separates the skin and fat layer from the muscles of the abdomen as far upwards as the ribs and frees the navel from its attachment to the skin. Stretched abdominal muscles are tightened if they are slack. The overhanging part of the skin and fat layer is removed and the wound is closed so that the tummy is as smooth as possible. The navel is sewn back into its usual position.

Sometimes a collection of fluid, blood or plasma, accumulates under the skin in the post operative period. It can usually be removed quite easily with a needle but this procedure may need to be repeated several times.

Areas of the skin can die sometimes as a result of infection or if there is a reduction of the blood supply to the edges of the wound. This may happen if the skin is pulled too tight or it can be a consequence of the patient's heavy smoking. If it results in wide scars they can be improved by scar revision later. Fortunately this complication is unusual.

The new navel may not be in the right place but it can be altered if necessary.

There will be an area above the long horizontal scar that will be numb. This results from the unavoidable damage to the sensory nerves that supply the area. These nerves regenerate slowly and after several months sensation begins to return.

The patient should stay slim as weight gain defeats the whole purpose of the operation. A regime of good diet and plenty of exercise will ensure that the result of the operation is permanent. The tummy will stretch again if the patient becomes pregnant, so this is an operation for women who have completed their families.

Abdominal lipectomy causes a permanent improved to the shape of the tummy if it was poor before the operation. It often encourages patients to adopt a healthier regime of diet and exercise because they look so much better. They may be able to wear clothes that they could not before and feel more confident in underclothes and on the beach.

COSMETIC SURGERY – A PERSONAL CHOICE

The decision to undergo Cosmetic Surgery is a very personal one.
So too is the choice of hospital.
Hillside Hospital in Ealing offers a complete professional service. Every stage, from initial assessment to surgery and beyond, is undertaken by Consultant Surgeons, assisted by fully trained staff.
For more information and a confidential assessment with a Consultant Surgeon, please telephone: 0800 616 220 (free of charge) or write to:
Hillside Hospital
Freepost (PAM 6804)
London W5 2BR
✣ Cosmetic Surgery   ✣ Plastic and Reconstructive Surgery   ✣ Dental Implantation

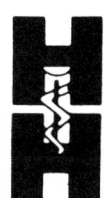

Hillside Hospital

22 Corfton Road, Ealing, London W5 2HT
Tel: 081-998 0045 Fax: 081-991 9525 Telex: 922172

VARICOSE VEINS

Varicose veins are veins which have become widened and at the same time more tortuous. They affect about 20% of the population of Great Britain, affecting women 4 times as often as men. There is an inherited tendency in about 40% of cases. The commonest predisposing factors are obesity and pregnancy. The condition slowly worsens. Treatment will depend on the severity of each case and can only be assessed at preoperative consultation with the surgeon.

Mild cases are suitable for day case surgery under local anaesthetic. Tiny stab incisions are made over the varicose veins and they are removed with special instruments. Because the incisions are tiny, sutures are unnecessary. Afterwards a pressure bandage is applied for one week. More severe or extensive cases may need a general anaesthetic. As well as removing the individual veins the groin vein is tied off via a small incision in the groin. The stay in the clinic is usually 1 or 2 days depending on the severity of the condition.

The tiny scars in the legs are hardly noticeable once they have matured.

There is often quite significant bruising and swelling but this usually resolves in a few days. Very rarely the bruising does not resolve completely leaving an area or areas of purple or blue discolouration.

Sometimes spider or thread veins appear in patients who are predisposed to them. It is impossible to predict which patients will develop this complication but those who already have areas of spider veins are more likely to suffer this effect. Spider veins can be treated with injections.

Occasionally a superficial sensory nerve can be damaged causing sensory changes. These symptoms resolve once the nerve has healed.

The individual veins which bothered the patient beforehand will be removed by the operation and they cannot return. However the tendency to develop varicose veins will still be present and further varicose veins will therefore appear in time. It is better to get these treated fairly regularly because treatment is then easier and more effective. The treatment described above gives an excellent cosmetic result and is better than injection treatment which is uncomfortable, cumbersome and antisocial for the patient and has a high recurrence rate because the injected veins can open up again.

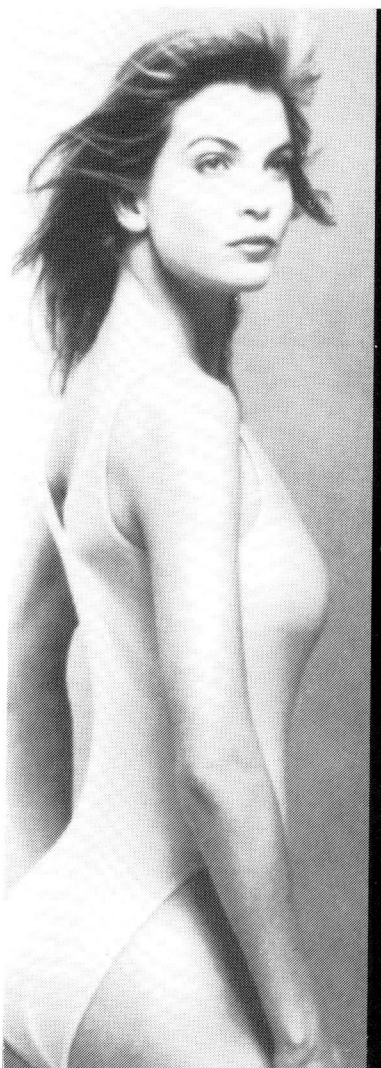

COSMETIC SURGERY

*f*or a consultation on ear, nose or abdominal reshaping, breast enlargement uplift or reduction, facelifts, eyelid surgery, varicose vein removal or spot fat removal (liposuction), call us on the number below or write for our colour brochure, video and further information.

A PRIVATE HOSPITAL ESTABLISHED OVER FORTY YEARS

West Hampstead —Clinic—
9 Hilltop Road London NW6 2QA

071-624 7366

CS86

Name:

Address:

Please send me further information on:

SPIDER OR THREAD VEINS

Thread veins are abnormally widened (dilated) small blood vessels very close to the surface of the skin. They most commonly occur on the face and legs and are usually inherited. They become more prominent with increasing age and can occur in clusters, especially on the face, causing patchy discolouration (redness). Thread veins are worsened by excessive exposure to the sun and wind and extremes of temperature. Alcohol makes them more prominent because it causes them to dilate more. Doctors do not know why some patients get them and others don't. In those who are predisposed to this irritating condition, any treatment of varicose veins, i.e. by injection or surgery, can exacerbate the appearance of thread veins in the legs.

Treatment may be by either electrolysis or by injection. Electrolysis involves applying a fine needle to the skin over the thread vein and passing a tiny electric current. This cauterizes the vessel and prevents blood from flowing through it, making it invisible. Electrolysis is best suited to the fine facial thread veins but not the large ones. The main disadvantage of electrolysis is that it can produce tiny pitted scars which are permanent. Sometimes a new crop of veins appears after a course of treatment. Injection treatment (sclerotherapy) is more suitable for the larger thread veins in the legs. Sclerosing fluid is injected directly into the thread vein by a very fine needle. The inflammation produced causes the walls of the vessel to stick together thereby preventing blood flow through it and making it invisible. Several injections may be necessary and recurrence is common.

Localized bruising, swelling and redness is common initially and this resolves within a few days. On rare occasions a brownish discolouration may occur at the injection site and take several months to fade.

The treatment is uncomfortable, not painful. Injections are performed on a walk in walk out basis with no dressing or bandages being required. Injections are carried out at two to four weekly intervals.

Dermabrasion will remove thread veins from the face but they would need to be very marked to justify this treatment.

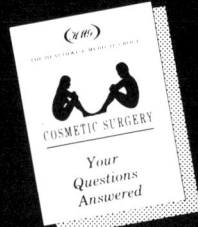

This *FREE* booklet tells you all you need to know about
COSMETIC SURGERY

Naturally you need reassurance about Cosmetic Surgery. So first of all send for our booklet.

It shows how our specialist surgeons use their outstanding skills to improve facial features, contour of the body, reduce fat, treat unsightly veins – and much more.

The Healthwise Medical Group can offer a no obligation consultation with surgeons of the highest calibre together with an all inclusive price package with no hidden extras.

THE HEALTHWISE MEDICAL GROUP
081-458 5728

618, Finchley Road, London NW11 7RR

Please send me details on: _____
Name. Mr./Mrs /Miss /Ms _____
Address _____
_____ Postcode _____

CSG

REMOVAL OF TATTOOS

Tattooing is the introduction of pigment under the skin to produce a permanent mark. Decorative tattoos are either self-inflicted or professionally performed. In the majority of cases young men have them put on as a result of bravado or peer pressure and later on they very much regret them, especially when they realise that tattoos are not accepted in society or often by employers. it is then that requests are made to have them removed. Unfortunately it is a lot more difficult to remove a tattoo than to put it on in the first place.

Surgical treatment is the only possible way of ensuring that all the pigment material is removed. If it is small, the tattoo can be totally excised and the resulting wound closed with stitches. The resulting scar being preferable to the tattoo. When the tattoo is large it cannot simply be cut out. If the depth of the injected pigment is not too deep, the surface of the skin can be removed by several methods such as dermabrasion, laser treatment or with a skin graft knife. If the pigment is deep in the skin the area may be excised and the defect covered with a skin graft.

The procedure can be performed under local or general anaesthesia depending on the size of the tattoo and the preference of the patient and surgeon.

Where the tattoo has been excised and the defect sutured the resulting scar may become stretched or thickened depending on the site of excision. Where a skin graft has been used there will always be a permanent mark. The grafted area will be a different colour compared to the surrounding skin and it will be hairless. Altered pigmentation as a result of sunburn may occur and the margins of the graft may become red and raised. In addition the graft donor site may not heal perfectly though in the majority of cases it heals well.

Generally regretted tattoos can be removed, but only at the expense of significant scarring in most cases.

COLLAGEN
REPLACEMENT THERAPY

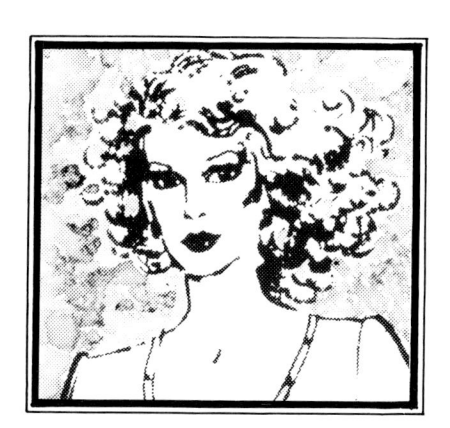

Established in 1984, MIRAGE is a company run by women for women, and is the U.K. leader in the use of Collagen Replacement Therapy. This non surgical treatment smoothes age lines away in minutes.

We offer friendly and helpful advice on all aspects of Collagen treatment and Aesthetic plastic surgery. We can arrange a **Free and Confidential** Consultation either in your own home or at your nearest Beauty Salon.

For more information, please call:
Midlands or North – Sally on 0455 556313
London, the South & South Wales – Marrianne on 071-249 3567

MIRAGE
MEDICAL GROUP

The White House, Kimcote, Leicestershire LE17 5RR

SCAR REVISION

Unsightly facial scars and blemishes can very often be improved by well planned and carefully executed surgery. A cosmetic surgeon cannot make invisible scars. He can only make the scars as inconspicuous as possible. The aim of scar revision is to achieve a scar which is fine, level and even with the surrounding tissue, about the same colour as the adjacent skin and which causes no pull on the surrounding structures.

The old unsightly scar has to be removed first. Any planned surgical incision heals in exactly the same manner as any other deliberate or accidental cut, i.e. it produces scar tissue that is nature's method of healing. Once an incision is made and sutured the surgeon has little control over the healing process, a fact that must be appreciated by the patient. A period of 6 to 18 months must elapse before the scar is mature, which is the stage where no further change or improvement will occur. Gentle massage with the fingers, using skin cream tends to improve scars during the maturation process.

Initially any scar will be red and raised above the level of the surrounding skin and may often be hard in consistency. Gradually the redness and hardness lessen and resolve leaving a soft scar which is level with and somewhat paler than the adjacent skin. For these reasons scar revision must not be undertaken too soon because adequate time must lapse to allow the healing tissues to mature.

When revising a scar on the face the surgeon attempts to get the best possible result by placing the new scars parallel to or actually in one of the normal crease lines of the face. This usually means that the direction and shape of the original scar has to be changed.

Excision of large scars or blemishes may require several operations over a period of time. Some areas of the body always produce noticeable scars e.g. nose, chin, chest, shoulders, upper back and parts of the arms and legs.

In summary therefore, the goal in scar revision is improvement and not perfection. Patients who are unable to accept this should not have treatment.

Most facial scars can be revised under local anaesthetisa. Extensive scarring in adults and scars in children are best treated under general anaesthetic. Most scar revision procedures can be treated on a day-care basis but some may require an overnight stay in the clinic. Dermabrasion is very effective for superficial scars on the face.

It is most unlikely that any scars can be removed completely, but the aim of the procedure is to make them less noticeable and perhaps easier to disguise with make-up.

THE TREATMENT OF BALDNESS

Surgery cannot give a man who is bald more hair. However the remaining hair can be surgically repositioned to cover the bald areas. Not everyone is suitable for surgery and each case must be carefully evaluated before a treatment programme is started. Every patient who contemplates embarking on a treatment programme must ensure that he is properly advised and fully understands the nature of the treatment as well as the probably outcome. Successful treatment of baldness depends on a number of factors: 1. The age of the patient and the amount of current hair loss. 2. The probably future loss of hair. 3. The quality and quantity of donor hair available. 4. The flexibility of the scalp. 5. The patient's expectations.

Surgical procedures currently include:
Male pattern baldness reduction Under local anaesthetic on a day-care basis part of the bald scalp is excised. The process is repeated until the small remaining bald area and the scar can be covered with hair using hair transplantation.

Hair transplantation Under local anaesthetic on a day-care basis, cylinders (plugs) of hair-bearing scalp are cut from the back and sides of the head and then placed in bald or thinning areas of the scalp. Several procedures are required to produce the effect of a full head of hair but the introduction of smaller grafts than were previously used has greatly enhanced the ability of the surgeon to produce a cosmetically pleasing result, without the tufted appearance which is associated in many people's minds with hair transplantation. The technique of hair transplantation is a relatively simple surgical procedure but it is difficult to get consistently good results because of the unpredictability of the various steps that are involved.

Skin flaps Hair-bearing skin flaps from the sides of the scalp can be rotated to cover the bald areas at the front.

A poor hair transplant looks worse to the patient than his original baldness. In the past many ruthless private clinics attempted to give too many people full heads of hair resulting in far too many disasters. Only a few people are actually suitable for hair transplantation. The remainder should be actively discouraged or at least try some of the effective scalp lotions available today. However there are many patients who have had extremely successful hair transplants and who are very pleased with their result.

Ointments and lotions Minoxidil was originally used as a drug to control blood pressure and it was soon discovered that it promoted hair growth. It is not known why it works but it undoubtedly does produce more hair in a small percentage of patients.

Antiandrogens are preparations which block the action of the male hormone, testosterone. Together with minoxidil, antiandrogens are being used orally and applied directly to the scalp. Results are still being evaluated.

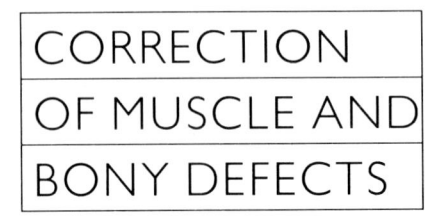

CORRECTION OF MUSCLE AND BONY DEFECTS

CALF AUGMENTATION

There are two types of patient who seek this operation. The first are those who have had an injury or a disease, such as polio, which has affected muscle development in one or both legs and where the patient wants the calves to be made normal or symmetrical. The other group consists of those who have normal legs but the calf region is too thin and the patient is embarrassed in clothes that show them. In both groups the treatment is essentially the same, which is to use an elongated soft silicone implant to plump out the affected part.

With the patient anaesthetized the surgeon creates a pocket over the affected muscle to accommodate the implant. As with breast augmentation the results are immediately obvious.

In patients with normal calves the result is usually symmetrical but in patients with a severe muscle defect in one leg it may not be possible to exactly match the other side with an implant.

Occasionally shooting pains and temporary loss of feeling can occur.

The most serious complication of this operation is deep venous thrombosis. It is rare. It is very important that patients should not be taking the pill and have stopped smoking for at least four weeks before the operation.

The operation boosts self-confidence because it stops people feeling embarrassed when wearing clothes which show the legs. It is also used by body-builders.

SUNKEN CHEST OR PECTUS ESCAVATUM

This is a condition where there is a large dent in the centre of the chest. It is more common in men. Sometimes the deformity is so severe that it affects breathing and these cases require thoracic surgery. Lesser cases are dealt with by filling the defect with a moulded silicone implant placed under the skin.

PECTORAL IMPLANTS

There has been a recent vogue amongst body-builders to have a specially shaped implant inserted underneath their own pectoral muscles to make them seem bigger. It is more commonly performed in America than here, where it has not really caught on. The incision is placed in the armpit. For many years pectoral implants have been used on just one side in the case where one of the pectoral muscles has failed to grow properly and does not match the other. The implant when used in this way does provide some improvement in symmetry but it cannot of course move in the same way that the ordinary muscle does. This is not a problem for the body-builders because the built-up muscle disguises the implant very effectively.

SKIN LUMPS AND BUMPS

Skin lumps are usually classified according to the tissue or cell of origin and whether they are benign or malignant. They are most commonly removed for cosmetic reasons. Sometimes it is necessary to remove them to treat, exclude or prevent malignancy. In addition lumps are removed for microscopic examination to establish a definite diagnosis where doubt exists.

TREATMENT

The treatment of any skin lump will depend on the diagnosis.

Benign skin lumps can be treated by surgical excision, shaving, electrocautery, cryosurgery, curettage, dermabrasion, laser as well as with topical chemicals in some cases.

For more information about skin lumps you should consult a surgeon.

WHY CINDY JACKSON HAD TWELVE OPERATIONS IN FOUR YEARS:

'MY FACE IS MY FORTUNE SIR', SHE SAID

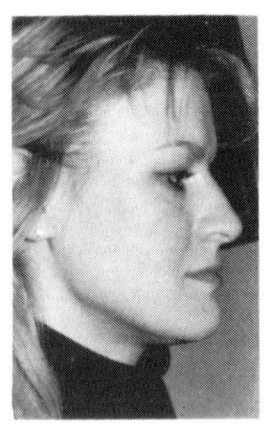

ORIGINAL PROFILE
(BEFORE ANY SURGERY)

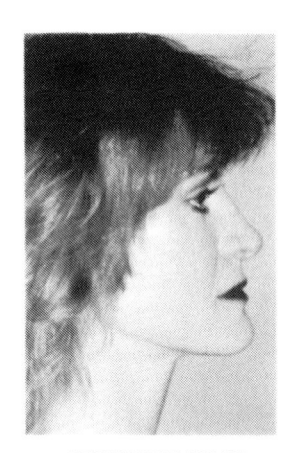

AFTER MY FIRST NOSE JOB

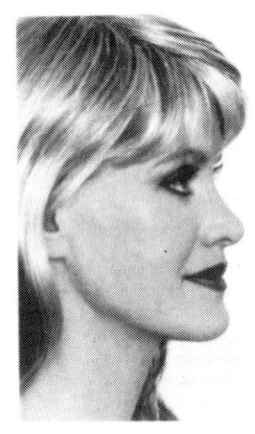

AFTER MY SECOND NOSE JOB
(BY A DIFFERENT SURGEON)
AND UPPER LIP OPERATION

These are the stunning 'before' and 'after' profiles of Cindy Jackson – the girl who would be pretty.

American-born Cindy was raised on a farm in 'Hicksville' USA. She was bright and ambitious but all she wanted was to be as pretty as her sister.

With more than a hint of irony when her father died she used £25,000 of the family money to 'get rid of the family resemblance'.

It was the start of a brand new life – Cindy began to remodel her features to look the way she wanted – the way she had always wanted.

She started with an operation to 'widen' her eyes, followed by liposuction on her chin, knees, thighs and abdomen. A lower facelift, silicone breast implants, two 'nose jobs', lower eye revision, a temple lift, upper lip enlargement plus a few other 'minor procedures' – completed the fairy tale story . . . Cindy was a new woman.

Now she wants to share the priceless knowledge gained from her own experiences with cosmetic surgery with other people who are thinking about 'going under the knife'.

The Cosmetic Surgery Network was launched in London in November 1991 – aimed at simply providing the public with vital information about cosmetic surgery procedures – information that isn't always easily accessible or available. "To the uninitiated the world of cosmetic surgery is a real jungle," she said.

"The network began as a way of communicating with people who contacted me following my regular appearances in the media – I was getting letters from people all over the world keen to hear about my own personal experiences with cosmetic surgery. I also made contact with those who had undergone surgery themselves and wanted to compare notes.

It soon became very clear that, while there was no shortage of doctors and surgeons for those seeking medical advice, there was a genuine and urgent need for information of a different kind to be made available.

So in response to popular demand I set up The Cosmetic Surgery Network – a private, independent and confidential information exchange."

The Network arms prospective patients with two types of information, which in all cases has been approved by a cosmetic surgeon:

1. Details of the procedure the patient is considering. These are from medical literature, but describe the operations in user friendly language.
2. CONSUMER REPORTS: Unique to The Cosmetic Surgery Network, these contain inside information not usually given to the public. There are also regular reports on new treatments and procedures. Cindy and her research committee share their findings of what really works, and what doesn't.

Added Cindy, "From Day One of setting up The Cosmetic Surgery Network, I have been inundated with detailed accounts of personal case histories of cosmetic surgery experiences of every description. Up-to-the-minute medical information is faxed to my office from what has now become a worldwide network of sources. I regularly meet with doctors and surgeons on both sides of the Atlantic, and I see hundreds of cosmetic surgery patients. As a result, I am now in the unique position of being able to maintain an ongoing cumulative view of the state of cosmetic surgery in Britain and abroad, in addition to the knowledge I gained through my own extensive research and firsthand experience. I am certainly not alone when I say that I wish I'd had access to more helpful information of this kind when I first started having cosmetic surgery back in 1988. I would have saved literally thousands of pounds and countless hours of research – and I would have gone about things very differently knowing what I know now. It is my aim to pass this knowledge on to others through The Cosmetic Surgery Network. If you are considering cosmetic surgery, you really should talk to me first!"

NB: The Cosmetic Surgery Network is a non-profit organisation and is NOT associated with any clinic that advertises. For further details, please send a large stamped addressed envelope to: The Cosmetic Surgery Network, P.O. Box 3410, London N6 4EE.

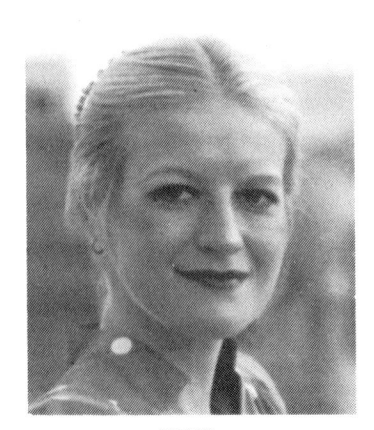

BEFORE

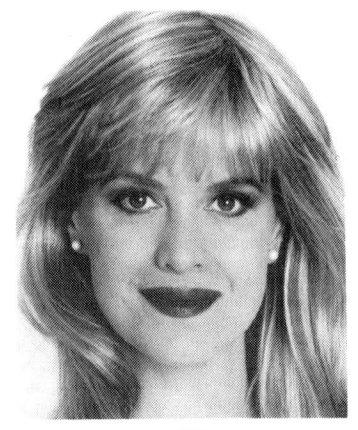

AFTER

SMILE
PLEASE

The British Dental Health Foundation outlines some of the latest dental techniques available today.

The perfect mouth. Rows of clean white healthy teeth in total symmetry.

And it's all within reach, thanks to modern dental technology. Those people whose teeth are less than perfect now have the chance to enhance what mother nature has provided. Dramatic advances in recent years have ensured that the dentistry business now really does have something to smile about.

Porcelain crowns, perfect bridgework, implants, magnetic dentures, veneers, inlays, onlays and braces – these are techniques widely available on the 'dental market' today.

Here we describe a sample of work Britain's dentists can offer patients in 1993.

FRONT TEETH WHITENING

A smile can be easily enhanbced with tooth coloured 'white' filling materials. Modern materials give such good results it is often quite impossible to 'see the join'.

A crown (or cap) may be necessary if a tooth is badly decayed or broken but smaller defects can be treated using methods which actually glue fillings to teeth. This is achieved by treating the tooth surface with special conditioners and then applying the adhesive. one advantage of this technique is that it can be done painlessly – sometimes without even having to numb the tooth first.

"Composite" filling materials can be moulded into the tooth's shape and then set by shining a special blue light. Alternatively, from a model of the tooth, a skilled dental technician can make a piece of shaped procelain which the dentist then bonds permanently in place on the tooth.

CHIPPED TEETH

o part of our body is stronger than our teeth but they are brittle and can be chipped. Large fractures need crowns but for lesser damage composite filling materials or porcelain are commonly used. Modern adhesives are now so advanced that it is possible in some cases to repair broken teeth simply by sticking them back together again.

THE GAP

A gap between two teeth can look attractive but sometimes closing the space can improve the smile. This can occasionally be achieved by wearing a brace (even with adults) or by using 'white' filling materials.

VENEERS

Unsightly visible front teeth surfaces (due to ageing, wear or discoloured fillings) can often be improved by covering all the showing surface with a veneer.

Just one visit to the dentist can transform a tooth by composite filling material being glued to the whole front surface. Alternatively if porcelain is used some tooth shaping will be required, and a mould taken. The veneer will then be made up at the dental laboratory. These veneers are very thin, like false finger-nails, but they are very strong and when bonded in place can be quite indistinguishable from a natural tooth.

FILLING BACK TEETH

Silver/grey amalgam has been the standard filling for back teeth for the past 150 years. Although strong and durable many people find this material unattractive.

Today there are two new tooth-coloured materials which are strong but look entirely natural.

These are Composite Filling Materials – colour matched and bonded to the tooth, and Glass Ionomer Cements. These are glass-like materials which can also be bonded to the tooth where some of its surface has been lost.

INLAYS AND ONLAYS

These are resin or porcelain-based and normally more expensive than fillings as they require considerable amounts of surgery time plus the use of a highly-skilled laboratory technician – but they do offer a more permanent, strong, life-like appearance. As 'onlays' they are used to replace biting surfaces which have been destroyed by grinding.

BRACES (orthodontics)

Orthodontics means the straightening of teeth which are crooked, crowded, jut out or tilt in. A brace is used to gently move the teeth into improved positions. This can take up to two years and although best results are achieved in childhood this technique is often used in adults with great success. The advantages are a nice even smile and an improvement in the outline of the face – occasionally speech too is improved by orthodontic care.

CROWNS (caps)

When a tooth is crowned it is shaped by the dentist while the patient has a local anaesthetic. Using a rubber-like material an impression is taken and sent to a dental laboratory for the crown to be made to the dentist's exact specifications of colour and shape.

It takes about two weeks to complete the procedure and during that time the patient will wear a temporary crown.

Crowns can be made of procelain or a metal alloy. The decision as to the best type depends on the position of the tooth in the mouth. If it's near the front then porcelain may be the material chosen. However, where the teeth are used to chew and grind at the back of the mouth then the alternative of the stronger porcelain bonded to metal is usually better.

Gold alloy is particularly suitable at the back of the mouth.

BRIDGES

If you lose a tooth you either need a denture or have some form of bridge constructed.

A dentist will make a conventional bridge by preparing the teeth on either side of the space as if they were to be crowned. Then at the laboratory two crowns are made with an additional tooth held between them. These bridges are made from gold and other alloys with bonded porcelain. They are fixed into the mouth using a quick-setting dental cement. Bridges can be small, replacing just one tooth or more complex, replacing a number of teeth.

Before any work of this type can be considered the gums around the supporting teeth must be in a really healthy condition.

Crown and bridge work is not cheap because of the time, materials and expertise involved – but some crowns and bridges are available under the National Health Service.

DENTURES

Dentures are important in replacing lost permanent teeth so you can enjoy a healthy diet and smile with confidence.

Historically many materials have been used to make dentures. Today dentists use the latest acrylics to produce lightweight but durable dentures. Metal-based dentures are made from stainless steel, gold or cast chromium cobalt. Before recommending the more expensive metal-based denture the dentist will have taken into consideration the strength of your bite and your wish to retain more taste sensation by having less of your palate covered.

Other denture variations include 'Swinglock Dentures', enabling the splinting together of loose teeth and the replacing of any missing natural teeth and – 'Magnetic Dentures'. Magnets are placed in the plastic denture base and in the top of retained roots. When the denture is placed over the roots magnetic forces keep it in place.

KEEPING YOUR TEETH HEALTHY AND LOOKING GOOD HAS NEVER BEEN EASIER

THE CHELSEA HARBOUR DENTAL PRACTICE PRIDES ITSELF IN PROVIDING ITS CLIENTS WITH ACCESS TO DENTISTRY'S MOST UP-TO-DATE DIAGNOSTIC AND COSMETIC SOLUTIONS CARRIED OUT IN A FRIENDLY, RELAXED ENVIRONMENT.

FOR A FREE OF CHARGE DENTAL ASSESSMENT AND BROCHURE DETAILING OUR SERVICES

Telephone 071-351 7931

NIGEL WEDGWOOD GRAVES B.D.S.

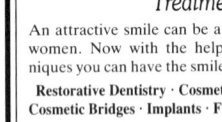

COSMETIC DENTISTRY

Treatment for Beautiful Teeth

An attractive smile can be a great asset for both men and women. Now with the help of advanced dentistry techniques you can have the smile you have always dreamed of.

Restorative Dentistry · Cosmetic Fillings · Porcelain Veneers
Cosmetic Bridges · Implants · Free initial consultation (not NHS)

KAREN LETH
DENTAL SURGEON – 071-631 0605
23 HARLEY STREET LONDON W1N 1DA

COSMETIC DENTISTRY

can change your life and improve your confidence. We can offer a variety of painless techniques. For further information call us now for a practice leaflet:

**Jonathan Portner & Associates, Dental Practice,
8–9 Thornfield Parade, Dollis Road, London NW7 1LN.
Tel: 081-349 3924.**

IMPLANTS

An implant is usually a metal device which is surgically embedded into the jawbone, leaving parts protruding through the gum – these act as an anchor for fitting a full or partial denture or even a crown.

Before any treatment the whole mouth must be brought up to a very high standard of hygiene. This is a very specialised technique and has only recently been introduced in Britain.

If you have a problem or need advice, write enclosing a self-addressed envelope to The British Dental Health Foundation, Eastlands Court, St Peter's Road, Rugby, Warwickshire CV21 3QP.

THE BEST PART OF 'BREAKIN UP' IS KNOWING HOW TO MAKE IT UP...

You don't need to be a £10,000 a day supermodel to look and feel good. If you follow these health and beauty guidelines you can quickly learn the secrets that make the 'stars' look great. We tell you how to create a pout as pretty as Naomi Campbell's, explain why apples and grapes are good for your face, why a simple plaster can help stop the frown lines, why aerobic exercise is so important, how you can give your hair new life and an instant 'high-wattage' shine and why vitamins can be your ACE in the pack . . .

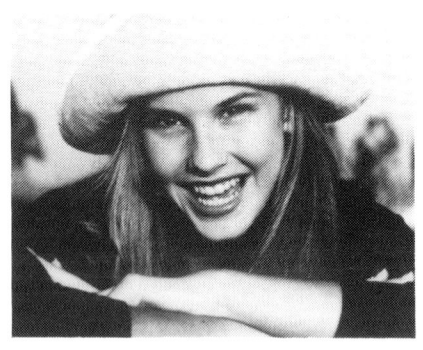

Shake Up Your Make-up

Every make-up artist knows that a successful make-up is about subtle changes and attention to detail. Often all you need is a touch of colour here or a little extra definition there.

The following professional tricks will ensure you make all the difference to your look, with the minimum of time and effort.

EASY BASICS

A good concealer is a must in every woman's make-up kit. Most make-up artists keep two shades for their own use, a lighter one to use on shadows under the eyes and a slightly darker one for when they have a slightly deeper colour, for instance in the summer months.

There are two good ways to apply concealer: either with a firm, flat brush, or by pressing a little on with the fingertips and then blending away.

You can also use concealer as an instant eye brightener. Brush or press a little concealer onto the upper lid as well as under the eyes. It will hide the purpley veins there and helps to give a much brighter, fresher look to your face.

Many women steer clear of foundation and powder, afraid that the colour match will be wrong, and/or look over made-up.

However, modern foundations and powders are so sheer and easy to apply that you won't look as if you are wearing make-up at all; and because they give just a fine veil of colour, you only need to apply them where you want them rather than all over.

The big beauty benefit of wearing a base is that shadows and blotchy areas are evened out, giving your skin a flawless finish. Powder will ensure that your make-up, including your blusher, stays just where you want it all day long.

Be sure to check how a foundation looks on your face out in the daylight before you buy it. Apply three shades that are closest to your own skin in strips next to each other, along the jawline at the side of your face. If you cannot find a shade that almost disappears on your complexion in that range, try another one.

Foundation-and-powder-in-one is a time-saving trick which also gives a super-natural, semi-matte finish. Simply use the cosmetic sponge provided to smooth the silky base all over your face; there is no need to apply additional powder on top. Professional make-up artists know that you don't want a skin to look completely matte and flat. With a very subtle sheen, such as these new compact foundations supply, the skin will look healthy and alive.

Alternatively, you can have foundations and powders custom-blended to perfectly match your skin. This service is available in department stores and some leading chemists countrywide.

CHEEK TO CHEEK

Blusher can look wonderful – or if you don't get it right, disastrous. The secret of choosing the right colour is to use a natural hue rather than a bright one and to follow the rule "less is more".

Team your blusher colour both with your own skin tone and your lipstick, and bear in mind the colour of the clothes you are wearing.

You can place your blusher in the prime position by smiling slightly and starting in the middle of the apple of the cheek, directly below the centre of your eye.

The fashionable look now is to keep the blusher in this central area to give the impression of rosy cheeks. Or you an follow the cheekbone up towards the outer corner of your eye, being careful not to take it as far as the hairline.

It is a smart move to replace the small brushes supplied in compacts with a large blusher brush of your own in order to create a more realistic effect.

Look out for the cream-and-powder mix blushers which are applied with a make-up sponge. They are good for the day as they give a soft flush to the cheeks.

LIP BOOSTERS

You can create a pout as pretty as supermodel Claudia Schiffer's or Naomi Campbell's. Apply a lip pencil just outside your natural lipline (but don't be tempted to go too far outside your own line!). Then fill in with a matching or slightly lighter lipcolour.

State-of-the-art lipsticks now contain micro particles which release their colour during the day with the natural movement of the lips, so providing a longer-lasting result. Many also have anti-ageing nutrients such as vitamin E and high-powered moisturisers.

A great way to enjoy wearing brighter colours is to use a translucent lipstick. These are not as slippery as glosses but still allow the texture of your own lips to show through.

SENSATIONAL EYES

Eyebrows are the frame for your entire face. Usually, the best place for them to start is from the point that lines up with the inner corner of the eye. They should run to just the outer edge of the eye. To check this, you can take a pencil and place it at an angle from the base of the nose to the outer part of the eye and up to the brow. The point where it crosses the brow is where it should finish.

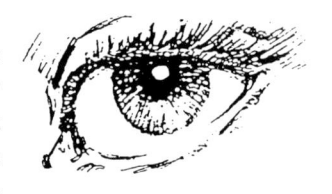

If you are going to pluck your eyebrows, pluck from underneath only. Try darkening them with eyebrown pencil or by applying a little clear mascara. You will notice immediately how your face takes more shape.

NAIL IT

Well-groomed hands and nails require just a little extra time. Keep a pump-action hand lotion by the sink and apply a little to both hands and nails every time you wash them.

Nails that tend to flake and peel are lacking in oil and moisture. Massage in a cuticle cream every night to help improve their condition and to prevent the hangnails that result from dryness.

Buffing the nails once or twice a week is a good way to improve the circulation and health of the nails as well as to boost shine.

EXERCISE – THE VITALITY FACTOR

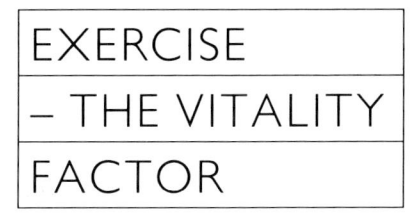

Exercise is the all-round body and mind improver. It helps you to make the most of your life by increasing your energy levels, it gives you a body that is toned and strong and it helps to keep your skin young by boosting circulation and oxygenation of the cells.

There are three types of movement that are key to the exercise equation:

Stamina + Strength + Flexibility = Fitness

Your weekly workouts should therefore include these three forms of exercise. You need to take aerobic exercise to increase your stamina and energy; do weight-bearing movements such as a gym workout to build the strength of both your muscles and bones; and include stretching exercises to balance your strength.

To help motivate yourself to take regular exercise consider the following health benefits:

- Aerobic exercise offers protection against cardiovascular disease.
- Weight-bearing exercise helps to prevent brittleness of the bones in later life (osteoporosis).
- It maintains good posture.
- Activity increases energy levels. If you don't exercise, even everyday tasks seem draining.
- Exercise raises your metabolic rate so that you burn calories more effectively even when you have finished your workout.
- Aerobic exercise has been scientifically shown to be mood-boosting and to be an effective way of fighting mild depression when compared to other forms of therapy. It releases beta-endorphins which deliver the feel-good factor.
- Exercise increases your self-esteem and body confidence.
- It gives you a great body!
- It is sociable and fun.

MAXIMUM RESULTS, MINIMUM TIME

It is much more beneficial to exercise for shorter periods every other day than to do a longer workout once a week.

When exercising you should allow a day in between sessions for your body to rest and repair, and so become stronger than before.

To achieve the cardiovascular improvements that vigorous (aerobic) exercise offers, you should do 20–40 minutes of aerobic exercise three of four times a week. Add some weight-training workouts in between.

Remember that exercising with weights does not need to build bulky muscles. By performing more repetitions with lighter weights, you will increase your muscle endurance.

When you are commencing an exercise programme, it will pay dividends in the long run if you begin with a fitness assessment. An expert will be able to draw up the right plan for you that will ensure your time is spent in the most productive areas.

Commit yourself to becoming fitter over a period of six weeks. After that, you should feel so much better than before that you will not drop out of your programme.

SKIN
SOLUTIONS

Skin care today is concerned much less with skin types than with providing solutions to problems as they arise.

Your skin condition probably changes frequently. Some days it may seem more sensitive, other days drier or oilier. Many women and men also find that they need to switch to different products with the changing seasons.

It is important to find a skincare regime that your skin responds well to and that can be adapted as required. New developments in formulations that protect against, and reduce the signs of, ageing are rapidly increasing in number.

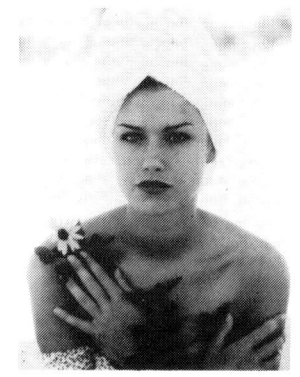

Let's look at the latest treatments and the benefits they may be able to offer you.

FRUIT ACID FACIALS

The latest breed of potions that claim to reduce the appearance of fine lines and wrinkles are called fruit acids or Alpha Hydroxy Acids (AHAs). Using extracts of fruits such as apples, grapes, lemon and passionfruit or, in some instances, sugar cane or lactic acid from milk, the acids are combined with moisturisers.

AHAs act like a gentle form of skin peel by increasing exfoliation and stimulating the turnover of new cells. Cosmetic companies say that it generally takes four to eight weeks for lines to diminish. Most women and men who try them find that their skin does develop a healthy-looking glow.

The effects are nowhere near as dramatic as those obtained with Retin-A (also known as tretinoin), the acne treatment which found popularity as a wrinkle treatment in recent years. Not officially approved as an anti-ageing treatment, Retin-A has been falling out of favour with cosmetic surgeons who have found that a high proportion of those using it suffer side-effects of dramatic reddening and scaling. The treatment must be maintained for life and you cannot expose your skin to the sun.

WATER THERAPY

Some companies believe that water is the secret of beautiful skin. They recommend cleansing the skin with a water-soluble cleanser, then rinsing it away by splashing the face up to 20 times. In some instances, the system uses water that is precisely at body temperature.

The principle is that the skin will be hydrated by the water which is then sealed in with a good moisturiser. Often the first step of the programme is cleansing with an oil which combines with the oils on your face, removed in the next stage by the wash-off cleanser.

It is a method that when used, with the right products, brings benefits to all skin conditions – dry, oil, combination or normal – helping to restore balance. It has been shown to be effective on acne skins.

ANTI-AGEING WORKOUTS

A number of skincare experts believe that much of what we perceive as skin ageing is, in fact, due to slackened facial muscles. By performing specific exercises every day we can both help to prevent the signs of ageing and correct them.

The exercises take perseverance to learn, but can bring dramatic improvements. Done correctly there should be no risk of stretching the skin which is one drawback that has been proposed.

MASSAGE AND AROMATHERAPY

Massage is one of the great skin boosters. Whether you do it yourself at home or have professional facials at a salon, massage will increase circulation, help to feed the cells and ease out lines of stress and tension.

There are a number of specialised massage techniques that can be bought as a course of skin rejuvenation. These use acupressure and other massage methods to bring results.

Many skincare products now contain essential oils from plants. These aromatherapy formulations are designed to relax, soothe, cleanse or moisturise the skin more effectively. Look out for ingredients such as rose geranium, chamomile, mallow, lavender and ylang-ylang.

EVERYDAY ULTRAVIOLET SCREENS

Dermatologists are now advising us to use moisturisers that contain ultraviolet screens every day, year-round. this strategy is designed to protect the skin from UVA rays which surround us all the time and pass through glass. The damage that these rays exact is believed by many experts to contribute strongly to premature ageing. Check that your facial moisturiser contains ultraviolet filters (the packaging may say 'broadspectrum ultraviolet filters' on the back). Increasingly body lotions and creams are also being formulated with UV protectors.

FROWN LINES

There are two treatments for frown lines that you can do at home. Exfoliating the area gently every day using a facial scrub will increase cell turnover. You can also train yourself to break the habit of frowning. By applying a specially shaped plaster, for instance overnight, you will unconsciously become aware of when you are frowning and so learn to stop yourself from doing so.

HAIR
REPAIR

Of all the aspects of your appearance, it is your hair that can make the biggest difference to your look.

Follow these top tips to ensure your hair is in peak condition and to make the most of your style.

- Always use the right shampoo and conditioner for your hair type. If you use a product for dry hair on greasy or fine hair, for instance, you will weigh it down and leave it looking dull.
- If you use styling products every day, a build up of residue from them can occur, making your hair look lifeless. Use a deep-cleansing shampoo that says it is formulated to combat build up.
- You can give your hair a high-wattage shine instantly with one of the new "laminators". These transparent silicone serums are applied to towel-dried or dry hair to smooth down the cuticle and reflect the light. They are great for short or long hair and can simply be applied to the ends.
- Colouring your hair can immediately visually enhance it. It can also be used to cover grey hair. There are now formulations which will hold for 6 weeks and effectively cover grey hair. These offer longer lasting effects than semi-permanents, which hold for up to 6 shampoos, without the commitment of a permanent change of colour.
- Very dry hair will benefit greatly from a professional deep-conditioning treatment. Protein is applied to the hair and heat-treated to help repair the damage. These treatments are more powerful than the deep conditioners you can use at home, which are very helpful when used once or twice a week.
- If you swim regularly, try to cover your hair with a hat to avoid the drying effects of chlorine. You should not expose chemically-treated hair (bleached, coloured or permed) to chlorinated water. Use a shampoo that will remove chlorine and follow up with a good conditioner if you do swim without a hat. Bleached hair can take on a green tint when it comes into contact with chlorine. You must seek the advice of a hairdresser if this occurs.
- Experiment with styling lotions. There are some which boost body, others which allow you to shape and style. If you blow dry your hair, look out for styling lotions that also protect your hair from heat.
- Hot brushes are a quick way to inject extra style into your hair as you dry it.

EAT TO WIN

You hold one of the most important keys for your day to day well-being and future health in your own hands.

Your diet has a powerful and direct action on how you feel. In fact, food is being hailed as nature's pharmacy. It has the ability to prevent degenerative disease or, in some cases, to contribute to it.

There are six nutrition strategies which, when followed consistently, will set you on the road to high level health.

1. IT'S ACE

Vitamins A, C and E play a protective role in the body, acting as anti-oxidants. Anti-oxidants neutralise "free radicals". These highly reactive molecules are the body's bad boys, causing ageing and disease. Studies are showing that these vitamins may be protective against cancer.

Make sure your diet is high in fruits and vegetables which contain the ACE protectors, such as carrots, citrus fruits, melon, blackcurrants and plums. Vegetables also supply important enzymes which have a powerful deactivating effect on cancer-causing agents. Broccoli, Brussels sprouts, cabbage, cauliflower and spinach are especially beneficial.

The added benefits of eating plenty of fruit and vegetables is that you will be eating a higher proportion of alkaline forming foods. Eating too many acid-forming foods can lead to calcium being withdrawn from the bones to counteract acidity, contributing to arthritis and osteoporosis in later life.

Increasing your intake of vitamin C after the exposure to the sun helps to protect against the sun's ultraviolet rays. Skin vitamin C levels are severely depleted after exposure, reported the British Journal of Dermatology.

2. OMEGA OILS

Oily fish such as salmon, mackerel and sardines are rich sources of the Omega 3 oil. Having just two fish meals a week can dramatically reduce your chances of ever suffering a heart attack. You will also increase resistance to other diseases and health problems including arthritis, breast cancer, eczema, migraine headaches and multiple sclerosis.

Fish oils have also been shown to be useful for pregnant women at risk of premature labour.

3. FABULOUS FIBRE

On average we eat 20g of fibre in the UK (vegetarians consume on average 42g). The minimum recommended intake is at least 30g per day. Lack of fibre is associated with increased incidence of diseases of the colon. Wholegrains, pulses, vegetables and fruit are all valuable sources of fibre.

4. FAT FACTS

The majority of us need to reduce our intake of saturated fats, while increasing our consumption of foods that contain monosaturated oils (olive oil), polyunsaturated oils and the EFAs – the essential fatty acids which are linoleic and linolenic acid.

Tossing a few sunflower seeds onto salads or on top of cereals and eating a few handfuls of fresh nuts a day provides adequate essential oils for the body.

5. GARLIC AND ONIONS

Experts believe half a clove of raw garlic every day may help to prevent heart attacks and strokes by increasing the body's blood-clot-dispersing activity. It also has antibiotic properties and boosts the immune system.

Onions boost the blood's good cholesterol for 3 out of 4 people and improves the blood in several ways. They are also considered a good all-round 'medicine', killing bacteria.

6. VITAL SUPPLEMENTS

Women of child-bearing age who may become pregnant are advised by the Government and nutrition experts to take a supplement of the B vitamin folic acid. This has been proven to prevent spina bifida. You should take a supplement of 400 mcg every day before conception and for the first 12 weeks of pregnancy.

BEAUTY CLINICS & SALONS

AMBER HEALTH and Beauty offers a positive, effective, up-to-date approach to Beauty Therapy. Specialised treatments include permanent lip-lining and eyebrows, Reflexology, eyelash perming, Thread vain removal, Aromatherapy, Backscratchers nails, Collagen replacement therapy. Shereday's Courtyard, 22 High Street, Billericay, Essex. Phone 0277-630952.

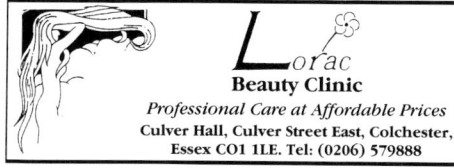

Lorac Beauty Clinic
Professional Care at Affordable Prices
Culver Hall, Culver Street East, Colchester, Essex CO1 1LE. Tel: (0206) 579888

JUNE NORMAN Beauty Clinic, Institute of Electrolysis MBABThC., MSBTh., AMIE., DRE. Est. 1976. Registered electrolygists, waxing, facials, broken veins, massage, ear piercing, etc. Incorporating E.R. Nail Studio, Elizabeth Ring D.R.E. Tel: Camberley (0276) 63615, Normandy House, 7 Prior Croft Close, Prior Road, Camberley, Surrey GU15 1DE.

CHRYSALIS BEAUTY SALON
PROFESSIONAL BEAUTY THERAPIST OFFERING EXTENSIVE RANGE OF BEAUTY TREATMENTS
★ Waxing ★ Facials ★ Eyebrow & Lash Treatments ★ Aromatherapy Massage
★ Make-up ★ Nail Treatments ★ Slimming Treatments ★ Specialist in Electrolysis & Red Veins
Hydro Lifting Complete Treatment, Skin-Peeling, Deep-Cleansing & Rejuvenating Facial
Fern Silvester HDBTH CGBTH, 61 Victoria Road, Ruislip Manor, Ruislip. Tel: (0895) 621422. 081 959 1999

STELLA GOODALL L.C.S.P.(B.Th.) Thread veins & skin tags removed. Advanced 'blend' electrolysis. Facial & body treatments, massage, steam, sauna. Arormatherapy, skin care. The Beauty Room, Church Road, Kessingland, Lowestoft (0502) 740427.

Panache   HAIR AND BEAUTY SALON
42 High Street Battle East Sussex TN33 0EE
SPECIALISTS IN RED VEIN TREATMENT, SKIN TAG REMOVAL & ELECTROLYSIS ALSO SLIMMING & MAKE-UP. COMPLETE TOP TO TOE TREATMENT RELAXING AND FRIENDLY ATMOSPHERE
Telephone: 0424 772801

MILO HAWKINS CLINIC, 24A Chertsey Street, Guildford, Surrey. Tel: 0483-60744. Slimming, universal contour wraps, beauty, Cathoiodermie, sunbeds, electrolysis, toning tables, aromatherapy, reflexology, skin and muscle tightening – Milolift. Treatments for Thread veins/warts moles and sclerotherapy.

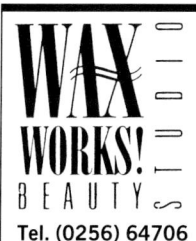

WAX WORKS! BEAUTY
Tel. (0256) 64706

Facial Red Vein Removal · Thread Vein Removal on Legs Using Sclarotherapy · Collagen Replacement for Facial Lines · Skin Peeling for Various Facial Complaints · Waxing · Arasys Inch Loss

We welcome your telephone inquiries or call in at
3 Potters Walk · Basingstoke · Hants

ACADEMY CLINIC – B.A.B.Th., C., M.S.H.B.Th. Established 20 years. Red veins treated on face and legs by Diathermy & Sclerotherapy, Electrolysis, facials, Aromatherapy & other beauty treatments. 56 Hawfinch Walk, Chelmsford, Essex. Tel: (0245) 266605.

PAMELA STEVENS Beauty Clinics offer the most professional and efficient beauty care for the discerning client. Tel: 071-700 1179 for details.

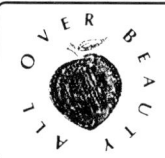

ALL OVER BEAUTY
FOR DETAILS OF OUR VAST RANGE OF BEAUTY TREATMENTS
TEL: (0284) 760191
6 GLASTONBURY ROAD
BURY ST EDMUNDS
Open 8am–8pm   Ample Parking

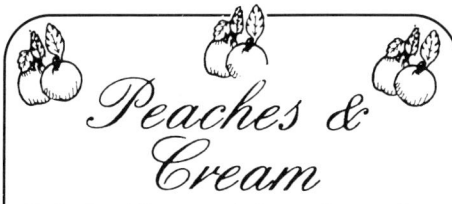

Peaches & Cream
Professional Treatment in Luxury Surroundings
● Fruit Acid Facial Peels ● Mini Health Farm Day ● Make-up lessons
● Collagen Injections ● Hair Salon ● Aromatherapy etc.
Tel: (0702) 75740
869 London Road, Opposite Chalkwell Park
Westcliff-on-Sea

FACE AND FORM is a charming beauty clinic, specialising in Thread vein treatments, Catiovital facials, Aromatherapy, Ionithermic for cellulite. Easy parking with friendly informed staff to make your visit a relaxing and pleasurable experience. Face and Form, 50 King Edward Rd, Abington, Northamptonshire NN1 5LU. Tel: 0604 35469.

COSMETIC SURGERY

Our comprehensive range of corrective procedures for women and men includes:

- Body, breast, face, nose and ear re-shaping
- Eyelid surgery
- Collagen replacement therapy
- Cellulite removal
- Varicose and thread vein removal
- Exclusive skincare treatment programme.

FOR A CONSULTATION WITHOUT CHARGE
PLEASE CALL YOUR NEAREST CLINIC

LONDON:	071-631 5494
MANCHESTER:	061-839 2527
BIRMINGHAM:	021-456 4334
BRIGHTON:	0273 324061

THE HARLEY MEDICAL GROUP
6 Harley Street, London W1N 1AA

SEE PAGES   FOR MORE INFORMATION

COLLAGEN

BATH, BRISTOL, CIRENCESTER, SWINDON, TAUNTON AND WESTON-SUPER-MARE
Collagen implants administered with care and gentleness by lady doctor.
For further information, please call
Cotswold Health Care on Bath (0225) 330948

YORKSHIRE   NORTHERN IRELAND

COLLAGEN REPLACEMENT THERAPY CARRIED OUT BY EXPERIENCED DOCTORS
HEALTHCARE 2000
Leeds (0532) 448866 Belfast (0232) 455556
Also: COSMETIC SURGERY & WEIGHT LOSS CLINICS

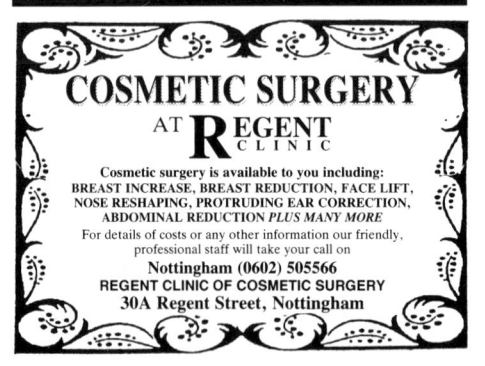

COSMETIC SURGERY

COSMETIC SURGERY
AT **REGENT CLINIC**
Cosmetic surgery is available to you including:
BREAST INCREASE, BREAST REDUCTION, FACE LIFT, NOSE RESHAPING, PROTRUDING EAR CORRECTION, ABDOMINAL REDUCTION *PLUS MANY MORE*
For details of costs or any other information our friendly, professional staff will take your call on
Nottingham (0602) 505566
REGENT CLINIC OF COSMETIC SURGERY
30A Regent Street, Nottingham

PRIVATE CLINICS

HIGHGATE PRIVATE HOSPITAL
PRIVATE ROOMS WITH EN SUITE FACILITIES
MODERN OPERATING THEATRES
Please contact Miss Maureen Reynolds for further information
081-341-4182

COSMETIC CLINIC

RUTLAND CLINIC
Professional Consultants For:
ADVICE ON SKIN CARE AND COSMETIC SURGERY
(INCLUDING THREAD VEIN TREATMENT)
Catering for Leics, Lincs, P'boro, N'hants and Beds
1A MARKET STREET, OAKHAM, LEICS
(0572) 770270

NON SURGICAL TREATMENTS

The Brentwood Medical Group
✻ Collagen Replacement Therapy
✻ Microsclerotherapy for thread veins
✻ M.D. FORMULATIONS, Glycolic acid product range/light peels ✻ Cosmetic surgery advice ✻ All treatments only by experienced medical practitioners
✻ Clinics in Harley St & Brentwood
BRENTWOOD MEDICAL GROUP
223 Coxtie Green Rd, Brentwood, Essex CM14 5RP Tel: 0277-375080
M25 Jct 28, 5 mins

COLLAGEN REPLACEMENT AND VEIN REMOVAL

Our doctors are expert in non-surgical treatment of facial lines using collagen replacement therapy and in the removal of thread veins.
Competitive skin management programme. Helping you look and feel years younger.
Visit our clinic in tranquil and relaxed surroundings near to M4, M40, M25.
Heritage HealthCare, The Pavilion Clinic, Plough Lane, Stoke Poges, Bucks SL2 4JW. ☎ 0753 662244

M.D. Formulations™

Now available in the UK direct from America M.D. FORMULATIONS the original AHA, Dermatologist developed "Fruit Acid" product range containing the key ingredient Glycolic Acid in concentrated form. This naturally occurring, non-toxic product is used in the treatment of FINE LINES, DRY SKIN, PIGMENTATION, AGE SPOTS, ACNE and SKIN SMOOTHING. HOME CARE PRODUCTS AND "LIGHT GLYCOLIC ACID PEELS"
Only available through doctors, private clinics, and trained beauty therapists.
For details of your local appointed clinic contact:
M.D. Formulations, Coppen Road, Selinas Lane, Dagenham, Essex RM8 1NU
Telephone: 081-592 1122

HAIR TREATMENT

An initial correct diagnosis & lifetime prognosis is absolutely essential in the treatment of hairloss, unfortunately few organisations realise this.

dhi

DHI INTERNATIONAL MEDICAL GROUP
37 Devonshire Place, London W1N 1PE
Tel: 071-224 1851

AN INITIAL correct diagnosis and lifetime prognosis is absolutely essential in the treatment of hair loss, unfortunately few organisations realise this. DHI International Medical Group, 37 Devonshire Place, London W1N 1PE. Tel: 071-224 1851.

HEALTH FARMS

CHAMPNEYS HEALTH Resort – superb sports and leisure facilities, extensive health and beauty treatments and deliciously healthy cuisine. Tel: 0442 863351.

RELAX IN the peace and quiet of a small residential country house Health Farm. All inclusive packages of diet & treatments. Brooklands Health Farm, Calderhouse Lane, Garstang, Nr Preston, Lancs PR3 1QB. Tel: 0995 605162.

HOAR CROSS HALL Health Spa. Resort in a stately home in Staffordshire. For more information call 0283 75671.

ROUNDELWOOD a Health Centre and Spa in beautiful Perthshire, Scotland combines a delightful holiday with superb treatments. Crieff (0764) 653806.

HENLOW GRANGE Health Farm, Henlow, Bedfordshire SG16 6DB. Tel: 0462 811111. A traditional health farm within 45 miles of London. 90 bedrooms, 180 staff.

INGLEWOOD Kintbury, Berkshire RG15 0SW. Britain's best loved residential health hydro. Top-to-toe. Days, 3, 4 and 7 day breaks. Tel: (0488) 682022 for brochure.

A caring and private environment with treatments, facilities and activities perfect for enjoying your recuperation.
GRAYSHOTT HALL, HEADLEY ROAD, GRAYSHOTT, SURREY GU26 6JJ.
Tel: 0428 604331

GRAYSHOTT HALL Health Fitness Retreat. A caring and private environment with treatments facilities and activities perfect for enjoying your recuperation. Grayshott Hall, Headley Road, Grayshott, Surrey GU26 6J. Tel: 0428 604331.

IMAGE CONSULTANCY

RITA READER Image Consultancy Service. Learn the rules of colour and line to enhance your colouring, minimise figure problems and achieve your ultimate attractiveness. Private consultations. Impersonalised colour analysis, make-up lessons, body line and wardrobe planning. Tel: 0268 758576.

PERSONAL GROOMING

PERSONAL IMAGE – ONE DAY GROOMING COURSE Colour/Figure Analysis, make-up, wardrobe plan, career dressing, confidence building, presentation skills, individual/corporate. Olivia Smith Image Consultancy (Hornchurch). Tel: 0708 446828.

RED VEINS, MOLES & WARTS

Red Veins, Moles & Warts
Expert removal of skin blemishes. Treatment of facial and leg veins... from £39.50. Permanent hair removal has been our speciality for nearly 60 years.
See your phone book for local clinic number.

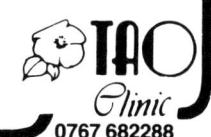

Aberdeen   Hull
Birmingham Liverpool
Cardiff   London
Carlisle   Newcastle
Edinburgh   Norwich
Exeter   Plymouth
Glasgow   Sheffield
Hatch End

TAO Clinic
0767 682288

SKIN CARE

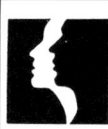

DERMACARE CLEAN SKIN
Clear skin with a safe, effective six day peeling treatment.
Over 50 years of success.
For free brochure telephone
081-766 7362.

TRAINING/COURSES

THE COLOUR COMPANY offers Certificated, Professional Training Programmes, Individual Consultations and Precision Dyed Colour Supplies for Independent Consultants within the Industry. Suzi Pickles, AMFIC, ITEC, Veryan, Vauxhall Lane, Southborough, Tunbridge Wells, Kent TN4 0XD. Tel: 0892 529474, Fax: 0892 517519.

BEAUTY SCHOOLS

LET BEAUTY be your future. Day and evening course leading to national and international qualifications. Send for free video. London Institute of Beauty Culture, 36 Dean Street, London W1V 5AP. Tel: 071-287 0474.